Disability Dialogues

Disability Dialogues

Advocacy, Science, and Prestige

in Postwar Clinical Professions

Andrew J. Hogan

JOHNS HOPKINS UNIVERSITY PRESS   BALTIMORE

© 2022 Johns Hopkins University Press
All rights reserved. Published 2022
Printed in the United States of America on acid-free paper
9 8 7 6 5 4 3 2 1

Johns Hopkins University Press
2715 North Charles Street
Baltimore, Maryland 21218
www.press.jhu.edu

Library of Congress Cataloging-in-Publication Data

Names: Hogan, Andrew J., 1984– author.
Title: Disability dialogues : advocacy, science, and prestige in postwar clinical
    professions / Andrew J. Hogan.
Description: Baltimore : Johns Hopkins University Press, 2022. | Includes
    bibliographical references and index.
Identifiers: LCCN 2022005146 | ISBN 9781421445335 (hardcover) | ISBN
    9781421445342 (ebook)
Subjects: LCSH: People with disabilities—United States—Social conditions—20th
    century | People with disabilities—Medical care—United States—History—20th
    century | Sociology of disability—United States—History—20th century.
Classification: LCC HV1553 .H65 2022 | DDC 362.40973—dc23/eng/20220302
LC record available at https://lccn.loc.gov/2022005146

A catalog record for this book is available from the British Library.

*Special discounts are available for bulk purchases of this book. For more information, please
contact Special Sales at specialsales@jh.edu.*

For Sabrina

Contents

Preface

Where are the disabled people in this history? What are disability communities' views of these events? Why have you chosen to freely interchange the terms *genetic disease* and *disability* here? As a late-stage graduate student, I found these incisive questions to be extremely jarring. Over the years, when presenting material from my dissertation and first book on late twentieth-century medical genetics, I was often asked to address disability perspectives on genetic testing and prenatal diagnosis. While I do not remember who most of my interrogators were, I am very grateful to them for speaking up and pushing me to think differently about the focus of my research. In all honesty, as a twenty-something, white, able-bodied man—who had a limited knowledge of disability scholarship and activism—I had not thought much about the relevance or impacts of my research on disability communities. As time went on, I increasingly came to appreciate that these were important questions—which I absolutely needed to address.

My colleagues' and audience members' consistent and welcomed encouragement was influential in my choice to center the advocacy and experiences of disabled people in my second book. Their probing questions led me to different conversations, which were ongoing in the historical background of my research area but had not received sufficient attention in my previous scholarship. Those who challenged me to reconsider my perspectives on disability introduced and engaged me in a new set of dialogues that altered and enhanced my worldview.

I have since learned that my own experiences were hardly unique. Disabled individuals and their allies have been asking pointed questions of researchers who too often overlooked or dismissed their perspectives for decades, pushing them to approach their topics in ways that gave greater voice and recognition to the experiences and perspectives of disability communities. *Disability Dialogues* explores the history of an ongoing "paradigm shift" in American society, toward viewing disability as a social construct, political identity, and valued form of diversity. I examine the impacts—real and potential—of these viewpoints on postwar clinical professionals.

In this book, I use the tools of a historian to make the case that the clinical professions need to do more to increase the representation of disabled people in their ranks. While new laws and the influential efforts of disability self-advocates have pushed clinical fields in this direction over the past half century, by and large clinical professions' concrete investments in recruiting and supporting disabled trainees and practitioners have been half-hearted and inconsistent, at best. Disabled people and their families have contributed significantly to the introduction and promotion of more positive, accepting, and sociopolitical narratives of disability in the clinical professions. Disabled clinical professionals are uniquely positioned to further these pursuits, by drawing from their biomedical expertise and their personal perspectives and experiences to help further break down resistance to more optimistic and accepting views of disability among their colleagues, students, and patients. Moves in this direction will be another major step forward in improving the inclusion, respect, and opportunities for disabled people in American society.

Acknowledgments

This project had multiple origin points. First, there were my many generous colleagues in the history of science and medicine who encouraged me to center disability in my historical analysis and helped me to think through the framework and focus of my research. Robin Scheffler, Nathaniel Comfort, Ruth Rand, Marion Schmidt, Susan Lindee, and Alexandra Stern were particularly important intellectual collaborators and influences. Then there was the archive. My entire summer of 2016 was spent on the top floor of the McGoogan Health Sciences Library at the University of Nebraska Medical Center working in the Wolf Wolfensberger Collection. Many thanks to archivists John Schleicher and Cameron Boettcher for their assistance and to my undergraduate research assistant Trevor Schlecht for helping me comb through Wolfensberger's numerous and eclectic materials and musings. Finally, there were all the clinicians and activists that I had the pleasure to interview for my first book and who, at the beginning of this new project, helped me to chart a course forward in examining evolving views of disability.

Several grants helped to get this study off the ground and provided support for the significant travel I did to archives and for conducting interviews. Initial funding was provided by the Center for Undergraduate Research and Scholarship (CURAS) and the Haddix Faculty Research Fund at Creighton University, as well as by a National Endowment for the Humanities summer stipend award. Significant support was then awarded by the National Science Foundation (#1655103) through its wonderful Science, Technology, and Society program. I also benefited greatly from a pre-tenure sabbatical in spring 2019, funded once again by the Haddix Faculty Research Fund at Creighton. These latter two awards made a huge difference in allowing me to complete much of my research by March 2020. Various grants also supported the twelve undergraduate research assistants who helped me on this project. I thank them for their many hours of productive, careful, and attentive work.

My disability-related research evolved along with my scholarly career, as

I moved from a PhD program in the history and sociology of science at the University of Pennsylvania, to the Science, Technology & Society Program at the University of Virginia, and for the past eight years as a faculty member in the Department of History at Creighton. My wonderful colleagues at all three universities have been influential and supportive of my work, in particular Adam Sundberg, Tracy Leavelle, Oge Williams, Heather Fryer, Kevin Estep, Molly McCarthy, Tom Svolos, Brooke Kowalke, Charise Alexander Adams, and Sabrina Danielsen. The Kingfisher Institute at Creighton has also been a valued intellectual home and funder of my efforts. I also want to especially thank Lynn Schneiderman and the rest of the Creighton University Libraries staff for helping me acquire countless important books and articles through interlibrary loan.

My findings and conclusions in this book were made possible by the collections of many archives. I greatly appreciate the ongoing assistance of Andy Harrison and Phoebe Letocha at the Johns Hopkins Chesney Archives, John Rees at the National Library of Medicine, Polina Ilieva at the University of California, San Francisco Archives, Lee Hiltzik at the Rockefeller Archive Center, and in particular to Elizabeth Deegan and Laura Labedz at the American Psychological Association, Susan Marshall and Allison Seagram at the American Academy of Pediatrics, and Virginia Corson for helping me to access a full run of the *Perspectives in Genetic Counseling* newsletter.

Interviews with clinical professionals and disability advocates were an extremely important, enjoyable, and informative aspect of my research for this book. I want to very heartily thank the 75 individuals who generously offered an hour or more of their time to speak with me about this history. Thank you in particular to the numerous disabled clinicians and activists and parent advocates who contributed so significantly to my research. A number of my interviewees provided valuable connections and resources. Some have also become my colleagues, trusted informal reviewers, and friends. Thanks in particular to Jon Weil, Virginia Corson, Robert Resta, Jack Stark, Barbara Biesecker, Bruce Shapiro, Stephanie Meredith, Erin Andrews, and Marsha Saxton. I was also honored and lucky to speak with many wonderful and influential people before they passed away, including Calvin Sia, Bruce Buehler, Marsha Saxton, and Murray Levine.

Many colleagues and friends in the history of science, medicine, and disability contributed their valuable time and input in shaping and improving this book. Thank you to Robin Scheffler, Henry Cowles, Stephen Casper,

David Law, and Jaipreet Virdi for reading early drafts of my manuscript, as well as to my anonymous reviewers. I also very much appreciate the opportunities that I have been given to present the material from this project at the University of Minnesota, the University of Oklahoma, Johns Hopkins University, and Weill Cornell Medicine's DeWitt Wallace Institute. The feedback and ideas that I received from the many participants in these forums were highly influential. Thanks to my many supporters in the academic community, who I have seen much too little of in recent years, especially Nathan Crowe, Jacob Steere-Williams, Kate Jirik, Jenna Healey, Courtney Thompson, Whitney Laemmli, Eli Anders, Julia Cummiskey, Pablo Gomez, Stephen Pemberton, Devon Stillwell, Janet Browne, Angela Creager, Theodore Porter, Naomi Rogers, David Wright, Sydney Halpern, Jeremy Greene, Mary Fissell, Elizabeth O'Brien, Susan Jones, Dorian Deshauer, Emer Lucey, Walton Schalick, Daniel Navon, Andrew Fenelon, and Beth Linker. I also want to thank Matthew McAdam, my editor at Johns Hopkins University Press, for championing this project and making it a priority for completion.

My family has been extremely helpful and influential throughout this project. Thanks to my parents, Pat and Gerry Hogan, for their continued inspiration and input and to my sister, Lauren Hogan, for all of our early and interesting conversations about this project. My wonderful son, Samuel Hogan, was born during the early stages of research and writing. Our always growing and changing relationship has offered me many needed opportunities for escape, reflection, and grounding, which have certainly improved the perspectives that I bring to this project. Finally, thank you so much to Sabrina Danielsen, my academic and life partner. Sabrina contributed in many ways by opening up the time and space needed to complete the research and writing for this book and always provided generous feedback on my ideas and writing as they developed.

Disability Dialogues

Introduction

Disability Advocacy in Postwar America

Mid-twentieth-century America viewed disability as a disruptive force. Clinical professionals were frequently called upon, or took it upon themselves, to intervene. Indeed, multiple post–World War II clinical professions owed their existence, prominence, or sudden growth to their established—and newly defined—roles in identifying, assessing, preventing, and ameliorating disability. During the 1940s, many politicians, scholars, and clinical professionals voiced concerns that soldiers returning home from war would be incapable of supporting themselves and their families, due to their physical and psychological wounds.[1] In response, the US government invested heavily in expanding the ranks of clinical psychologists to assist veterans in coping with newly acquired disabilities and fulfilling their anticipated social roles.[2]

Meanwhile, clinicians in other fields warned that children with intellectual and developmental disabilities caused families great stress—and led to their unraveling. Postwar psychiatrists and pediatricians took the lead in diagnosing these children early and encouraging institutionalization in many cases, to "protect" marriages and siblings.[3] More broadly, clinical professionals often presented people with intellectual and developmental disabilities as tragic and hopeless cases, who would be unproductive workers and drain social resources. Postwar genetic counselors worked to identify families at risk for having disabled children before they were born. The field grew quickly in the late twentieth century, as it helped to implement prenatal testing for the detection and prevention of disability—by way of selective abortion.[4]

Prominent disability scholar and self-advocate Harlan Hahn has argued that many people feel both aesthetic and existential anxiety toward disabled individuals. This has often led America's able-bodied majority to fear and shun atypical bodies and behaviors—due to their sense of revulsion, as well as discomfort with the reality that they too could one day be disabled. For many years, laws, policies, and social norms were in place to keep visibly disabled children and adults off the streets, away from community events and organizations, and out of schools, workplaces, and professional careers, by way of social marginalization and removal in residential institutions.[5] Postwar clinicians played key roles in justifying and implementing this exclusion, through their cultural authority to diagnose, prognose, and recommend approaches to management.[6] These ambitions were embedded in the identity and purpose of many clinical fields to prevent disability if possible and to isolate and ameliorate disability when necessary.

Overview and Aims

Disability is a historically and culturally relative concept, the meanings and implications of which are in constant flux. Throughout the postwar period (a general term I use in this book to describe clinical fields between 1945 and the present), new categories and conceptions of disability were adopted and expanded in social, clinical, and governmental settings. Along with these categories, terminology and diagnostic thresholds constantly evolved.[7] In the late twentieth century, many disability advocates espoused person-first language to displace dismissive labels such as "cerebral palsied child" in favor of placing the whole person ahead of the disability. More recently, disability self-advocates have increasingly embraced identity-first language, such as "disabled person," because it highlights the role of an unaccommodating society in actively disabling people. This construction also emphasizes disabled peoples' valuable and powerful social identity and political agency.[8] Mindful of these preferences, I limit my use of person-first language to more medicalized terms, as in a person with spina bifida or developmental disabilities.

Self-identifying as a disabled person can be a very personal and intentional choice, as well as a means of claiming participation in specific communities, political movements, and social programs. Many people cannot avoid being categorized as "disabled," especially those with visible differences. Others have been perceived or made to feel as if they had a disability only in certain environments. Some have found that they are able to "pass" as not disabled in some situations or periods of life but have chosen not to—for both personal and political reasons. Indeed, to be a disabled person has frequently been an important personal and group identity. One's disability status could be at once imposed, embraced, stigmatized, and celebrated. Many disabled people have sought to be viewed and addressed as part of a large demographic population and identity, akin to other minority groups in their history of marginalization and mistreatment but also in possessing diverse and valued cultures and experiences.[9]

Depending on one's perspective and social context, being seen as a disabled person could be a positive identity, a background consideration, or an unwelcomed imposition. At times, clinical professionals played a key role in shaping these statuses. Many disability self-advocates were very aware of, and often resisted, clinicians' power and oversight—seeking more influence and control over their own disability identity.[10] In addition, disabled people, like many other late twentieth-century activists in the clinical arena, sought to free themselves from medical paternalism, which limited their autonomy and access to social and clinical interventions.[11]

In parallel with the efforts and successes of civil rights movements driven by Black Americans and women during the 1960s and '70s, disability self-advocates pushed for the greater societal and legal inclusion of disabled people in the late twentieth century. These campaigns targeted many similar types of discrimination, which drew on essentialist assumptions about biological, social, and cultural inferiority, as well as the desire to maintain existing white, able-bodied, male-dominated power hierarchies, which denied equal access to public spaces, voting rights, educational institutions, and career opportunities.[12] The ongoing perpetuation of these inequities is rooted in physical spaces, as well as social and legal structures, institutions, and attitudes. They have been intermittently addressed since the 1950s, leading to significant but incomplete and variable advancements in challenging racist, sexist, and ableist discrimination. These exclusionary practices also impacted scientific and medical careers, which for much of the twentieth century were largely closed to women, racial and ethnic minorities, and disabled people. Various institutions made efforts to increase the inclusion of marginalized populations in biomedicine, but representation among most of these groups remained very low into the 2020s.[13]

Many scholars have described the post-1950 role of families, legislation, popular culture, and disability self-advocates in driving advances in acceptance and accommodations for disabled people.[14] Much less attention has been given to the influence of these trends on the training, research, perceptions, and practices of clinical professionals. In this book, I specifically examine the evolving medical and sociopolitical engagement of three clinical professions—clinical psychology, pediatrics, and genetic counseling—with disability and disability-related advocacy.

This is a history replete with unanticipated inspiration and strong-willed advocacy, as well as pessimism and reluctant responses from clinicians. Disability scholars have long lamented that disabled people are often presented as sick, tragic, or needy figures, rather than as dynamic and influential actors in historical accounts of clinical practice.[15] In this book, I situate disabled individuals and their families in clinical and community settings—importantly *not* just as patients and dependents but primarily as professionals, consumers, and advocates.

A small, but vocal contingent of postwar clinicians, including many who had visible disabilities themselves or disabled family members, took on powerful sociopolitical disability advocacy roles. They were at the forefront of introducing and promoting more positive and accepting views of disability in clinical training, research, and practice. With a few notable exceptions, historians have overlooked the significant contributions of these clinicians.[16] This book offers many accounts of postwar clinicians' relationships with disabled people, to analyze the role of personal encounters and experiences in encouraging new clinical perspectives.

Advocacy had various meanings for clinical professionals and disabled people, which fell into two largely distinct categories: (1) helping individual patients and families to navigate clinical settings and to identify community-based resources, and (2) promoting more accepting and sociopolitical perspectives on disability to patients and in the broader society. Most postwar clinicians felt comfortable with the former but avoided the latter, viewing sociopolitical disability advocacy as outside of their clinical domain and expertise. That said, many clinical professionals *did* engage in certain forms of sociopolitical advocacy—such as genetic counselors supporting abortion rights—but very few were actively involved in disability-related campaigns.

This book also highlights the influential activism of postwar *disability self-advocates*—disabled people who promoted more positive and inclusive disability-related policies and perspectives. While some self-advocates spoke up primarily for their own interests—or those of close colleagues or students—much of the self-advocacy that I describe addressed the shared goals and concerns of many and diverse disability communities. It is important to distinguish self-advocates from parent, family, and professional advocates, in part because members of these latter groups frequently maintained paternalistic doubts about the potential and influence of advocacy efforts that were developed and led primarily by disabled people.[17] As I demonstrate, many disability self-advocates strongly and effectively challenged these dismissals.

Even amid powerful advocacy efforts, the potential for postwar clinicians to adopt new narratives of disability was diminished by professional factors, which shaped clinical training, careers, ambitions, and institutions. In this book, I argue that clinical professionals resisted adopting more positive, accepting, and sociopolitical perspectives on disability in large part due to their concerns about professional role, identity, and prestige. Certainly, the commonplace aesthetic and existential anxieties associated with disabled people that Harlan Hahn described prejudiced some clinicians' personal views, and these attitudes cannot be neatly disentangled from their related professional interests.[18] Nonetheless, as I highlight, clinicians often perceived alternate perspectives, which characterized disability in terms of political and environmental factors, as challenging the priority of their practices and scientific ways of knowing. Many felt that such changes in perspective threatened their professional status and jurisdiction, as well as their preferred theories and approaches to measuring, understanding, and addressing disability.

Approaches and Concepts

Scholars of recent American history have benefited from access to a wide variety and wealth of primary sources. My narrative and analysis in this book rely on the examination and comparison of archival records, published articles and textbooks, professional newsletters, and about 75 oral history interviews with clinical professionals, disabled clinicians, and disability self-advocates. I use these sources to explore how clinical professionals responded to new laws, cultural changes, and advocacy around disability issues. Drawing from these records, I demonstrate the ways in which more positive and inclusive views and approaches to disability came into conflict with long-standing professional norms, concepts, priorities, and practices.

I came to this project from a background in the history of science and medicine. Much of this book's empirical content aligns with the scholarship in these fields—focusing on the structures and interests of scientific and medical institutions as well as their professionalization processes. That said, my larger ambitions for this book were shaped by the goals of disability history—to reveal modes of ableist oppression in our society and to highlight the many ways in which disabled activists, family advocates, and other allies have strategized and succeeded in countering discriminatory interpretations and enhancing the well-being and opportunities of disabled people. I hope that the hybrid orientation of this book allows it to meaningfully contribute to each of the often-divergent literatures of medical and disability history, but I also recognize that my approach may leave scholars in both fields feeling less than satisfied.

As a historian, I believe that it is important for me to use the terms of my historical actors, while remaining mindful that some of these words are offensive and harmful to disabled people. Clear descriptions and precise analyses of change over time are not possible without invoking the terminology of specific periods, in part because newer designations are not necessarily synonymous with historical categories. Also, there is significant historical relevance in conveying the evolving names of disability-related organizations, including the National Association for Retarded Children (NARC)—now The Arc; the American Association on Mental Deficiency; and the Association for the Severely Handicapped—later exclusively called TASH. Throughout this book, I carefully and intentionally use the words and categories of clinicians to achieve the most accurate characterizations of the past and ongoing evolution toward the present.

Postwar clinical professionals across many fields responded to disability advocates' promotion of new concepts and narratives with great reluctance. My examination of clinical psychology, pediatrics, and genetic counseling shows that the specific nature and implications of clinicians' considerations varied somewhat by discipline, due to factors including field size, degree type, relative status in the clinical hierarchy, and scientific commitments. Each of these variables informed clinicians' concerns about their professional role, identity, and prestige.

I address *role* primarily in terms of practice—what activities were considered necessary and appropriate (or dubious), as well as the primary contexts in which practitioners worked. For instance, genetic counselors highlighted their role as patient educators within clinical settings. *Identity* is related to a field's self-conception and ambitions—postwar pediatricians viewed themselves as uniquely qualified to be team leaders and sought after these positions. *Prestige* is associated with markers of status that individual practitioners could accrue during their career, as well as how other clinical professionals viewed their field. Many clinical psychologists saw the preeminence of their quantitative scientific measures as important to maintaining their prestige.

Role, identity, and prestige were often intertwined. Clinicians' desired roles and adopted identity were influenced by their perceptions of relative prestige. Professional jurisdiction was one area where all three intersected. Claims of jurisdiction—for conditions, patient populations, or service locations—had significant implications for clinical fields. Institutional recognition of jurisdiction could affect decisions about approving new medical subspecialties and certification boards, as well as how state governments chose to distribute funding. Sociologist Andrew Abbott defined jurisdictions as areas of exclusive social control through which one professional field could preempt competitors' claims. Abbott noted that jurisdictions were often established and kept exclusive through the development and mastery of abstract knowledge, like causal theories and treatments.[19] Postwar clinicians made jurisdictional claims over particular roles and practice locations, used jurisdictional designations to establish an identity as leaders in a specific domain, and viewed jurisdictional control as an important marker of career and disciplinary prestige.

Postwar clinical professionals viewed disability as a diverse category, which included many forms of physical, sensory, cognitive, and behavioral differences. Thus, there were many jurisdictional claims to be made over disability services, knowledge, and research. In this book, I address clinicians' evolving responses to many forms of disability, but I most consistently focus on intellectual and developmental disabilities. These conditions originated in childhood, were frequently associated with genetic causes, and commonly involved both physical and cognitive traits, making them potentially highly relevant to each of the disciplines I examine. Nonetheless, while some postwar clinicians identified intellectual and developmental disabilities as their specialty, this was a patient population that most others preferred to avoid.

The US government codified the term *developmental disabilities* in 1970, as part of expanding planning and facilities programs that initially targeted intellectual disabilities. Over time, the scope of developmental disabilities was expanded to include autism, dyslexia, and certain physical impairments originating before age 22. Developmental disabilities were not addressed as diseases to be cured or handicaps that could be overcome with rehabilitation but as chronic conditions that disrupted development and were likely to have lifelong consequences for self-care, learning, mobility, or self-sufficiency.[20] Notably, since much of postwar medicine was focused on preventing and "curing" acute conditions, or assisting people to overcome and adjust to newly acquired physical disabilities, mid-twentieth-century clinicians often marginalized, demeaned, or ignored research, training, and service on intellectual and developmental disabilities.

Evolving Approaches to Disability

During the first two decades after World War II, societal and clinical views of disability—and in particular developmental disabilities—were overwhelmingly negative and frequently nihilistic. Many physicians recommended immediate and lifelong institutionalization for children diagnosed with developmental disabilities. In hospitals, newborn disabled children were sometimes left to die in unseen wards and on outdoor balconies due to the hopeless attitudes of physicians and parents. Disabled children were viewed as a drain on society and as a potential threat to their families and communities. Parents who did raise disabled children at home were often excluded from public education and ostracized from social organizations and activities.[21]

Some families responded to stigmatization and exclusion by forming advocacy organizations, such as NARC in 1953. Through NARC, parents of children with intellectual and developmental disabilities fought for the same social resources and inclusion afforded to other, predominantly white, "ordinary, middle-class American families." Many NARC members challenged clinicians' assumptions that immediate institutionalization best served children's and families' interests.[22] Nonetheless, the population of children with developmental disabilities in residential institutions continued to grow in the 1950s and '60s, even as the population of psychiatric facilities was swiftly declining.[23] Eventually, disability advocates and journalists worked surreptitiously to reveal the horrific conditions inside large residential institutions for children with developmental disabilities. Their reports elicited widespread calls for change in the early 1970s.[24] From there, deinstitutionalization took place on a state-by-state basis. Along with it, clinical services for children with developmental disabilities were moved into community facilities, and parents gained greater influence in their fight for access to new social resources.[25]

During the 1960s and '70s, disability self-advocates drew on the rhetoric and successes of the civil rights movement to argue for equal access to education and other public spaces and resources. Beginning in 1962 at the University of California, Berkeley, Ed Roberts led a battle for inclusion and accommodations on college campuses for wheelchair users and other physically disabled people.[26] Later that decade, the Architectural Barriers Act (1968) required that buildings constructed by the US federal government, or leased with federal funds, be made accessible to disabled people. Parents of disabled children also fought for greater access to public education. In 1975, the US Congress passed the Education for All Handicapped Children Act (PL 94-142, later renamed the IDEA Act). This revolutionary law guaranteed free and appropriate education to all children, independent of their functional limitations and intellectual abilities.[27]

Despite legislative gains, many clinical professionals and members of the general public still viewed disability primarily as an individual deficiency, which had pathological origins and tragic impacts.[28] In response, disabled individuals and their families, along with other advocates, introduced new perspectives on life with disabilities. These alternative narratives provided more optimistic and inclusive views of disabled people and highlighted their unique experiences and contributions to their families and society. Also, rather than highlighting individual bodily deficits, advocates presented disability as resulting from social, environment, and institutional attitudes and barriers, which stigmatized disabled people and prevented them from becoming full members of society.[29] While medical conceptions of disabled people called for efforts to treat and rehabilitate the body, a new generation of sociopolitical perspectives on disability pointed to the need for societal changes to make communities more supportive, navigable, and accepting.[30]

During the closing decades of the twentieth century, many historically marginalized groups engaged in health and political activism.[31] In the disability arena, such self-advocacy was fundamental to achieving legislative and policymaking victories. A defining moment in postwar disability history occurred in April 1977, when self-advocates organized nationwide protests demanding the implementation of Section 504 of the Rehabilitation Act, which had been passed four years earlier. Section 504 mandated that the US government, as well as federally funded schools, institutions, and employers no longer discriminate on the basis of disability for access, employment, or education. These successful protests brought increased attention and momentum to the self-advocacy movement for disability rights, which continued to gain strength.[32]

A decade later, disability self-advocates played a major role in writing and campaigning for the Americans with Disabilities Act (ADA, 1990). These efforts included the "Capitol crawl," in which physically disabled individuals struggled to climb up the US Capitol's front steps to demonstrate continued barriers to access. The ADA extended protections and accommodations for disabled people in the labor market, education, and across all public spaces, including transportation.[33] During this period, disabled people also became more visible in popular culture, including the television show *Life Goes On* (1989–1993) starring Chris Burke, an actor with Down syndrome. By 2000, the social, cultural, and legislative achievements of disability advocacy were significant. Disabled Americans were increasingly being viewed and treated as equal and valued members of society, and yet their inclusion remained painfully incomplete.[34]

New laws did not translate into concrete gains for many disabled people in the early twenty-first century. Poverty rates remained disproportionately high for disabled individuals; their earnings were significantly below average; and their labor market participation continuously declined from its peak in the late 1980s. Disabled people who did achieve career success also faced challenges in building wealth and pursuing opportunities while retaining access to needed societal supports—forcing some to turn down job offers and professional grants. Many others found that they had little hope for any sort of career advancement.[35]

Disabled people continue to be very poorly represented in all clinical professions. While many fields sought to address their lack of practitioners from other marginalized groups, it was uncommon for disabled individuals to be actively included.[36] Intersectionality between disability and race has also been largely overlooked or underappreciated throughout much of disability scholarship. Disability history has primarily focused on white stories and activists.[37] My book, with its focus on postwar clinical professions that had very low representation among disabled racial and ethnic minorities, also fails to significantly address intersectionality between disability and race. This is an important topic, which I have begun to study for future publications.

Clinical Interpretations of Disability

Late-twentieth-century trends toward greater social, cultural, and legal acceptance and accommodations for disabled people influenced clinical reforms as well. In the 1970s and '80s, advocacy and media attention on cases in which parents and physicians allowed newborns with Down syndrome to slowly die of dehydration in neonatal units—instead of undergoing a simple, life-saving gastro-intestinal surgery—led to political and public backlash. Eventually, pressure from the Reagan Administration and amendments to the federal Child Abuse Act of 1974 brought changes in hospital policies and ethical perspectives. By the mid-1980s, the withholding of effective medical interventions for newborns with developmental disabilities had largely been abandoned. During this period, new surgical interventions were developed that could correct fatal heart anomalies, which were common in Down syndrome. Physicians' widespread uptake of these procedures greatly increased the life expectancy of children with this condition.[38]

Countervailing trends also emerged, especially as developmental disabilities were increasingly associated with specific genetic markers. In some cases, this led to the potential for prenatal genetic diagnosis and the option of selective abortion.[39] Many disability self-advocates emphasized that the widespread promotion and use of these techniques to prevent disabilities had negative impacts on people who presently lived with disabilities by reifying commonplace assumptions that life with such conditions was dreadful and not worth living.[40] The decision to prevent disability through abortion was left to women. Disability self-advocates questioned whether couples had sufficient and properly balanced information about life with certain disabilities to make fully informed choices, especially because they knew that many clinicians painted an overly pathological, grim, and hopeless picture of these conditions.[41]

Many disability advocates viewed prenatal diagnosis as a search-and-destroy mission, which sought to eradicate the atypical but valuable experiences and perspectives of disabled people.[42] They pushed clinicians to learn more about life with disabilities outside of the clinic, to put families in contact with advocacy organizations after diagnosis, and to be more sensitive and optimistic when speaking about the potential of disabled people and their families.[43] To counter overly narrow and negative clinical narratives, Rayna Rapp and Faye Ginsburg argued for the proliferation of "unnatural histories," of disability, providing "visions of lives lived against the grain of the normalcy."[44] Families facing prenatal choices about having a child with some form of disability benefited from realistic views of the path forward—of a life they could imagine pursuing, even if it was not what they had anticipated. However, most late twentieth-century clinical professional graduate programs were not offering these perspectives to their trainees.

Meanwhile, the interdisciplinary field of bioethics strongly influenced late twentieth-century clinical views of disability. Bioethical concerns during this period often centered on the distribution of scarce resources like organ transplants, dialysis, and other life-saving procedures. When bioethicists were called upon to assess and resolve these difficult issues, they often privileged their own conceptions of quality of life and acceptable functionality. Using these metrics, bioethicists frequently addressed disabled peoples' lives as less valuable and less worth saving. Disability self-advocates, as they sought to counteract pessimistic and tragic assumptions about disability, were highly critical of these judgments, which nonetheless held significant sway in clinical decision-making.[45] This book addresses multiple disability-related debates that drew the attention of bioethicists. In particular, I critique the long-standing practice in bioethics of seeking to "draw lines" that would ethically or objectively delineate "severe" forms of disability.

While bioethics has played a dominant role in shaping societal and medical views of disability, the experiences and advocacy efforts of disabled people who trained in and pursued clinical professional careers have received little scholarly attention. Historically, few individuals with outward or publicly acknowledged disabilities sought training in clinical fields. This has been due to stigma, dissuasion, and doubt on the part of their mentors and the gatekeepers in clinical training programs, as well as long-standing distrust and distaste for clinical professionals within disability communities. Beginning in the late 1970s, the US Rehabilitation Act prohibited the automatic exclusion of qualified people who had disabilities from clinical training programs. Academic studies over the subsequent decades pointed to the demonstrable success of people with physical and sensory disabilities in their clinical training activities and subsequent careers.[46]

After the ADA passed in 1990, more in-depth research identified some of the challenges that disabled clinical trainees encountered in arranging accommodations at clinical training sites, choosing a welcoming clinical specialty, and achieving ongoing career advancement.[47] Cognizant of these difficulties, many disabled clinical professionals have sought to highlight the valuable insights and diversity of experiences that they offer as trainees and practitioners. Disability self-advocates Tom Shakespeare, Liza Iezzoni, and Nora Groce have argued, "Perhaps the most dramatic learning can come when it is a peer who is disabled, rather than a patient. . . . [T]here is a need to open up admissions procedures so that suitably qualified people with disabilities can become health professionals."[48] Indeed, a powerful way to counter negative assumptions about disability among clinicians is to include and support more disabled people in clinical professional careers—as students, practitioners, researchers, teachers, and role models.

Social and Medical Models of Disability

Academic studies of disability in society have proliferated over the past half century. One of the most dominant and influential social science approaches to studying disability highlights distinctive and conflicting medical and social models.[49] Scholars have generally characterized the "medical model" as viewing disability as a bodily deficit or condition, which has a biological cause, and originates within an individual person. This framing leads disability to be viewed primarily as a health problem, affecting individual functionality and quality of life, which is best managed with biomedical interventions. Disability scholars and self-advocates established the alternative "social model" of disability in the 1980s.[50] Social model proponents view disability as the result of social stigma and insufficient societal supports, which oppresses people with certain impairments, making them disabled. The social model locates the causes of disability in societal decisions, structures, and marginalization, rather than individual bodily impairments, and calls for social, cultural, and environmental reforms. Importantly, social model advocates view disability primarily as a political issue rather than a discrete health problem.[51]

Historians of medicine have frequently pointed to the "medical model" as if it were a neutral term describing a conscious and widely embraced model of practice. However, the so-called medical model has rarely been identified or defended by clinicians as a representative professional philosophy, or as an intentional set of approaches for clinical training and practice. Instead, the term has been mobilized almost exclusively as a critique of clinical practice, either by clinicians arguing for reform or by disability scholars and other social critics in calling for the exclusion of certain disability-related or mental health issues from the medical domain.[52]

Undoubtedly, there has been rhetorical and practical value for advocates in contrasting "medical model" and "social model" views of disability. However, historical, social, and political analyses that draw on a bifurcated "social versus medical model" framing may unnecessarily perpetuate existing polarization and tensions between clinical and disability communities. In this book, I take a different approach. Instead of presuming that clinical professionals resisted new, more positive, inclusive, and sociopolitically oriented perspectives about disabled people due primarily to a medical model allegiance, I examine the various professional concerns, motivations, and pressures that influenced many clinicians' resistance to the social model and other alternative views of disability. In doing so, I reveal the ways in which considerations about professional role, identity, and prestige, along with preferred methodologies and ways of knowing, shaped clinical professionals' reluctance to adopt new disability narratives.

Many scholars have expressed discontent about "social versus medical model" framing, and some have suggested alternative analytic approaches. The World Health Organization's (WHO) *International Classification of Functioning, Disability, and Health* (2001) argued for a "biopsychosocial model," which integrated social, psychological, environmental, and biomedical aspects of disability. This perspective, which was coined by physician George Engel in his own 1970s-era medical model critique, viewed disability as a result of the interaction between a person and their social and physical environment.[53] Some disability scholars and self-advocates have criticized the hybrid approach of the biopsychosocial model, arguing that it emphasizes the health aspects of disability over political considerations. These critics presented the biopsychosocial model as simply an expansion of the medical model, which undermined social model perspectives by continuing to locate the origins of disability in individual bodily deficits.[54]

Certain aspects and assumptions of the social model have also been critiqued from within the disability community. Liz Crow and other disability scholars argued that the social model's focus on the abstract and constructed nature of disability too often overlooked the lived experiences of disabled people—particularly those with degenerative conditions or chronic pain. Even if disability discrimination ended tomorrow, Crow noted, some people with impairments would still benefit from medical interventions to improve their well-being. Indeed, all people, including those with disabilities, occasionally require medical assistance and benefit from a positive, trusting, and empathetic relationship with clinical professionals.[55] Historians of medicine have only recently begun to explore the importance of variable experiences of disability, in part by distinguishing "healthy" and "unhealthy disabled" populations. Importantly, this area of scholarship must speak to the widest possible range of disability experiences and should not be unduly focused on highlighting the most stable and nondisruptive forms.[56]

There has also been a push since the 1990s, driven in large part by disabled clinical professionals, to highlight the value of disability identity, culture, and pride. This "diversity model" perspective has sought to build upon and improve the social model by bringing disability experiences—including the impacts of impairment on daily life—back to the forefront in disability scholarship and advocacy. Disabled rehabilitation psychologist Erin Andrews and colleagues have argued that rehabilitation specialists like themselves, and clinical professionals generally, should help to introduce and encourage their patients to adopt a disability identity.[57]

Scholars in science and technology studies (STS) have similarly sought to highlight more diverse views of disability, by identifying the ways in which disabled individuals complicate and hybridize the implications of social and medical perspectives. Gail Landsman has explored how mothers of disabled children selectively *integrate* various aspects of both social and medical model perspectives—after finding neither viewpoint to be sufficient on its own. Along similar lines, Laura Mauldin has examined the ways in which hearing mothers engaged in "ambivalent medicalization" around the uptake of cochlear implants for their deaf children by simultaneously recognizing the benefits, challenges, and shortcomings of medical interventions. Mauldin has also highlighted the ways in which learning to hear with cochlear implants need not be seen exclusively as a rejection of sign language and Deaf culture but rather as an individual means of opening up "new modes of being deaf." Landsman, Mauldin, and other STS scholars have sought to look beyond ideological divides to focus on the lived experiences of disabled people and their complex interactions with various clinical and disability communities.[58]

This book builds upon scholarly approaches that have sought to overcome dichotomous perspectives and narratives—like the "social versus medical model" divide—with the goal of encouraging more complex, representative, multifaceted, and productive accounts of disability. I demonstrate how polarizing responses to new views of disability among clinical practitioners prevented productive collaboration toward achieving common goals, and led to professional concerns competing with the consideration of more sociopolitical approaches.

Outline of Chapters

This book is organized into two parts. The first three chapters (1–3) address the general postwar history of each clinical discipline and its evolving engagement with disability self-advocacy and family advocacy. Three additional chapters (4–6) examine specific case studies involving each field as its practitioners considered more positive, inclusive, and sociopolitical perspectives and approaches to understanding and managing disabled people against the background of concerns and pressures related to professional role, identity, and prestige.

Chapter 1 explores the powerful self-advocacy of multiple postwar disabled clinical psychologists, who pushed for more supportive, accepting, sociopolitical, and identity-based views of disability within their discipline. I highlight efforts in psychology to situate disabled people as a minority group and to celebrate their diverse experiences. This chapter also considers the disruptive divisions that often separated out advocacy related to physical versus intellectual disabilities.

In chapter 2, I examine campaigns to increase pediatricians' interest in research, training, and service involving children with developmental disabilities. During the 1960s, pediatrician Robert Cooke and Eunice Kennedy Shriver, who each had disabled family members, helped to facilitate the creation of new professional pathways, bringing greater prestige to the area. In response, pediatricians sought a more extensive leadership role for themselves in developmental disabilities but found that competing interests and financial constraints limited their influence.

Chapter 3 explores the contested history of clinical and community-based disability advocacy in genetic counseling. Most late twentieth-century genetic counselors presented their professional role and identity as expert and empathetic patient educators and advocates within clinical settings. A small cohort within the field pushed for more optimistic, inclusive, and sociopolitical views and advocacy around disability. I trace the influential efforts of these genetic counselors in developing more disability-positive and community-engaged training programs.

The next three chapters examine resistance and barriers to new disability perspectives, and their historical and structural basis in professional factors and concerns. Postwar science and medicine were not set up in ways that readily facilitated the adoption of more positive views of disability. Such transitions challenged professional identity, traditional ways of knowing, and methods, meaning that reform efforts could threaten prestige and career advancement. Clinicians were protective of their epistemologies, professional roles, and outcome measures—which were contested by new views on the nature of disability and the potential of disabled individuals.

In chapter 4, I examine disagreements in postwar clinical psychology concerning diagnosis and interventions related to intellectual and developmental disabilities. I examine efforts by advocacy groups, including TASH, to end the use of painful "aversive" interventions to alter atypical and potentially harmful behaviors, as well as new approaches to classifying intellectual disabilities and debates about the clinical validity and implications of facilitated communication. These episodes each reveal tensions that arose among clinical psychologists when more positive and inclusive views of disability conflicted with their scientific identities and ways of knowing.

In chapter 5, I describe competing efforts to claim ownership over the area of child development in postwar pediatrics, and how these debates intersected with practitioners' differing levels of interest and understandings about children with developmental disabilities. One faction focused on more "severe" developmental disabilities and viewed these conditions primarily as a result of organic brain damage. Another highlighted psychosocial considerations and support needs for children with more common developmental and behavioral conditions. Efforts toward collaboration between these areas were continuously disrupted by concerns about clinical jurisdiction and closely related professional considerations of role, identity, and prestige.

In chapter 6, I investigate the contested area of prenatal diagnosis and disability rights in the field of genetic counseling. During the 1990s, several disability scholars and self-advocates encouraged genetic counselors to adopt more positive and accepting narratives of disability in the prenatal context. While a few genetic counselors were receptive to their concerns, many practitioners in the field, along with its national association, resisted change. I highlight the importance of ongoing open conversations between genetic counselors and self-advocates in keeping the field engaged with disability issues. This proved especially important in the 2010s against the background of new technological advances and pro-life political advocacy efforts.

The epilogue builds on these two sets of histories to make a larger argument about the importance of encouraging and supporting more disabled people to pursue and thrive in careers as clinical professionals. Despite the legal and social changes of the past half century, there has been little increase in the representation of disabled practitioners among the clinical fields studied in this book.[59] In this chapter, I consider ways in which disabled clinicians might help to further enhance the uptake of more positive and accepting views about the lives, potentials, and contributions of disabled individuals, as well as the unique value of their experiential knowledge.

Clinical Psychology

Evolving Disability Perspectives and Advocacy

In August 1992, clinical psychologist Alice L. Riger expressed her disappointment with the American Psychological Association's (APA) level of engagement on disability issues for practicing psychologists. In a letter to the APA Office on Ethics, she wrote, "A number of disabled psychologists, including myself, would like to see APA taking an active, public, pro-disability rights stand, as we do in favor of minorities of gender, race, ethnicity, and sexual orientation. The Ethics Committee should be instrumental in insuring that otherwise qualified persons with disabilities receive equal opportunity within our profession."[1] Riger argued that APA should address the marginalization of disabled trainees and practitioners in psychology by showing the same level of concern and intervention as they did in instances of gender and racial discrimination. As part of this, she called for the accreditation of psychology training programs to be dependent on their disability access and accommodations, so that any qualified person could enroll and succeed. Later that year, in APA's professional magazine the *Monitor*, Riger posed the question, "Would APA allow racists to physically bar African-Americans at an APA-accredited doctoral program? Unlikely. But APA accredits doctoral programs that unfairly bar wheelchair users by being inaccessible or that refuse to accommodate other disabilities."[2]

Riger was one of numerous disabled psychologists in postwar America who called on their professional organization to be more welcoming and supportive of their diverse perspectives and needs. Many were inspired by the "minority group" conception of disabled people, which was first developed in the late 1940s by a small contingent of psychologists to help understand and explain disability discrimination in their profession and society.

These psychologists argued that many of the problems that disabled people experienced were not primarily caused by their individual impairments but rather by the stigma and misconceptions of the "non-handicapped majority."[3] Although this recognition was an important first step toward improved accommodations in the late 1940s, adequately countering the origins and impacts of disability discrimination within and beyond the psychology profession was a high bar, which Riger and others believed had not yet been adequately achieved nearly a half century later.

Psychology in late twentieth-century America was a large and diverse discipline, which comprised—and to some degree tolerated—a wide variety of epistemological perspectives and methodological approaches. Psychologists were trained and worked in a multitude of specialty areas and professional settings, including inpatient and outpatient clinics, academic departments, clinical and animal laboratories, schools, and private office practices. After World War II, the psychology discipline and APA came to be increasingly dominated by clinicians. This boom in clinical psychology was driven in large part by the US government's investment in training more PhD-level practitioners to address the mental health needs of returning veterans.[4]

I focus here on three professional groupings of postwar clinical psychologists: disabled psychologists, rehabilitation psychologists, and practitioners who specialized in intellectual disabilities. As I describe, there were frequent overlaps in the first two categories but a significant divide between them and the intellectual disabilities area. Most postwar rehabilitation psychologists worked in clinical settings with patients who had acquired physical disabilities. While a few also worked in the area of intellectual disabilities, this focus remained largely on the periphery of the rehabilitation field.[5] The same could be said of disabled psychologists—many of these practitioners had physical disabilities and specialized in rehabilitation, but almost none pursued research, service, or advocacy involving people with intellectual disabilities. Some rehabilitation psychologists lamented that disability-related topics had been relegated to their specialty and ignored by the rest of psychology.[6] In doing so, however, they overlooked the broad interest of other psychologists in intellectual disabilities. Indeed, many postwar specialties contributed to research, services, and training related to intellectual disabilities, including clinical, behaviorist, developmental, and school psychologists.

While rehabilitation psychologists and specialists in intellectual disabilities focused on different forms of disability and distinct patient populations, they did share in common an individual-level orientation. Postwar psychologists in general tended to privilege assessment, interventions, and experimental studies on isolated individual characteristics, deficits, behaviors, and responses—to the exclusion of larger social dynamics. Kurt Danziger has described mid-twentieth-century American psychology as "dominated by an individualistic social ontology" and noted the field's tendency to address "abstract individuals as objects of research." Likewise, prominent postwar psychologist Seymour Sarason often referred to the psychology discipline's perspectives, research methods, and theories as "asocial" and individual-focused.[7] These broader tendencies strongly influenced postwar clinical psychologists' conceptions and approaches to disabled people and made them more reluctant to consider sociopolitical perspectives on the causes and potential solutions to disability status, stigma, discrimination, and oppression.

Meanwhile, societal and professional issues related to disability rarely surfaced as significant considerations for most postwar psychology practitioners and trainees. Many graduate training programs in psychology barely touched on disability, and disabled psychologists often felt like marked outsiders at their professional conferences and places of work.[8] While APA established a track record of promoting racial and gender diversity during the postwar period, disabled psychologists often argued that they were included in such efforts often in name only and rarely through concrete, transformative actions. Amid this, many disabled practitioners encouraged colleagues to recognize their biases and complicity in disability discrimination and called on them to engage in making change rather than passively accepting the status quo.[9]

This chapter examines how various strains of postwar psychology—including Lewinian, rehabilitation, normalization, and positive approaches—informed the discipline's evolving views on disability. As part of this, I explore the important role of disabled psychologists in promoting more optimistic, inclusive, and sociopolitical narratives of disability in their field. I argue that many postwar clinical psychologists resisted calls to consider these novel perspectives on disability, and to promote reform in their profession and society more broadly, because they viewed disability as being caused by individual-level deficits, which were best treated with targeted interventions. Similarly, psychologists often addressed disability discrimination as the product of individual bad actors rather than institutional oppression.

Throughout the postwar period, disability advocates from a variety of specialties within psychology pushed for major changes in their field. These proponents of new approaches to disability held many views and goals in common. As I describe later in the chapter, due largely to a social and professional hierarchy in disability interpretations which privileged physical over cognitive disabilities, little engagement or collaboration took place between psychologists who specialized in physical versus intellectual and developmental disabilities. This situation disrupted the potential for broader political advocacy into the 2020s.

Psychological Aspects of Physical Disabilities: A Lewinian Approach

In the mid-1940s, the United States–based Social Science Research Council (SSRC) approached Stanford University psychologist Roger G. Barker about conducting a study of existing research on the psychological effects of physical handicaps—and specifically how this literature related to the potential problems of returning veterans. After receiving his PhD in 1934, Barker had spent two years at the University of Iowa working with prominent social psychologist Kurt Lewin and his assistant Tamara Dembo. Lewin was a Nazi-era German émigré, whose unique approaches to psychology—privileging person-environment interactions and real-world applications—briefly gained significant attention in the United States during World War II and up until his sudden death in 1947. The environmental orientation of Lewinian psychology represented a major break from mainstream research in the US and Germany, which focused on individuals in clinical or laboratory isolation.[10] Barker and Dembo, along with Beatrice Wright, another Lewin protégé, went on to strongly influence the specialty of rehabilitation psychology in America.

To complete the SSRC study on the social psychology of physique and disability, Barker recruited Dembo, Wright, and Lee Meyerson, a psychology PhD student at Stanford. In 1946, Barker and colleagues published *Adjustment to Physical Handicap and Illness*, which examined psychological responses to disability from a Lewinian perspective—rooted in the interactions between persons with and without disabilities and their environment. Meyerson later suggested that the report introduced a new theoretical perspective, which was the origin point for viewing disabled people as experiencing an "underprivileged minority status," akin to that of racial minorities.[11]

This "minority group" perspective on disability was more explicitly developed as part of a 1948 special issue on the social psychology of disability in APA's *Journal of Social Issues* (JSI). Barker proposed the collection and asked Meyerson to recruit relevant articles. By this time, Meyerson had been deaf for about half of his life. He sought out contributors who he believed might help to push the professional conversation and norms around disability in new directions. This included challenging the assumption that most disabled children could not go to public school due to their physical impairments and raising awareness about how negative terminology shaped individual, public, and professional perceptions of disability.[12]

In his introduction to the special issue, Meyerson highlighted the importance of the minority group view of disability as an expansive, testable, and sophisticated new theory. He explained, "Perhaps one reason why so much research in disability is of a trivial, molecular nature on the level of personality inventories, and so many conclusions are stated in terms of common stereotypes, is the lack of a guiding theory to indicate meaningful questions and define them precisely." Drawing on Lewinian themes, Meyerson criticized psychology's tendency to describe and understand disability as an essential characteristic of individuals rather than exploring the impacts of dynamic environmental factors and barriers. He hoped the special issue would help to generate more new theories on disability that looked beyond individual deficits.[13]

The next 30 years saw major social progress toward acknowledging and addressing discrimination against women and racial minorities in the United States, through legislation and changing societal attitudes. Many members of APA Division 9 on the Psychological Study of Social Issues (APA has 54 specialty and interest-based divisions, which function as societies within the association[14]) were inspired by Lewin's push for an "applied" social psychology. These psychologists contributed to major political transformations, for instance by offering testimony to the US Supreme Court in *Brown v. Board of Education* (1954).[15] Over the coming decades, race-based civil rights advanced, and the women's movement made progress in raising awareness about the discriminatory power of language. Meyerson, who became a prominent leader in late twentieth-century rehabilitation psychology (APA Division 22), had hoped to see similar achievements in overcoming disability-related discrimination but was ultimately disappointed.

During the 1970s and '80s, disability self-advocates led protests that successfully pushed for the enactment of Section 504 of the US Rehabilitation Act of 1973, while efforts to call out and replace stigmatizing terms like "crippled," "retarded," and "handicapped" began to gain traction. Amid all of this, however, APA Division 9 and JSI—its official publication—remained on the sidelines. Meyerson noted in 1988 that *no* subsequent JSI article had cited anything from the 1948 special issue on the social psychology of disability. In fact, only one JSI article—written by Tamara Dembo—directly addressed disability during this period. Responding to a 1985 survey, less than 1 percent of Division 9 members (5 out of 850) identified physical impairment as a relevant social issue.[16]

As postwar psychologists increasingly embraced civil rights and social integration, disabled people were rarely included in their thinking or efforts. In 1970, social psychologist and disability advocate Bernard Kutner lamented, "The disabled are not given the privilege of wearing the badge of their status with pride. Flaunting a disability is not considered acceptable. Thus, to paraphrase an expression, 'crippled is not beautiful.'"[17] Much of society continued to associate disability with tragedy or shame. Postwar social and clinical psychologists did little to acknowledge or address this ongoing discrimination. Even those who did recognize the significant impacts of disability discrimination made minimal efforts and expressed little hope about changing the status quo. For their part, most rehabilitation psychologists maintained their focus on researching and facilitating individual-level adjustment, coping, and acceptance.[18]

Dembo approached disability differently. She was one of the strongest voices within social and rehabilitation psychology advocating for an approach that put the discriminatory viewpoints and actions of nondisabled people at the center of psychological examinations of disability, as well as considerations about how to achieve societal change. In 1964, Dembo argued for the importance of recognizing the differing perspectives of "insiders" (disabled people and their close associates) and "outsiders" (clinicians and other nonhandicapped people) in rehabilitation psychology theory and practice. This standpoint theory on disability destabilized the traditional unidirectional relationship between "expert" providers and the presumed "neediness" and unreasonable expectations of disabled people and their families.[19] Insider/outsider framing was an early step in shifting rehabilitation psychologists' view of disabled people from being patients in need of "objective" information and professional help to actively engaged consumers. Dembo emphasized that disabled people and their families offered unique and valuable "insider" experiential knowledge of living with disabilities to professionals. This included viewing disability as a part, but not the totality, of one's identity and concerns.[20]

Drawing on her many years of work with Lewin, Dembo espoused the view that disability was a relational construct, rather than an individual characteristic. In 1973, she and her colleagues wrote, "In general, then, restrictions and handicaps are not only inherent in the loss or lack of properties of the person, but are in larger part due to the feelings and behavior of *other* people and to the rules and regulations of the outside world, the environment surrounding the handicapped person." Promoting a minority group perspective on disability, Dembo argued that the world was built *by* and *for* nonhandicapped people. Thus, it was the majority who held the power to maintain or change the status quo. Rehabilitation psychologists, she and her colleagues argued, had a legitimate role to play in promoting laws and policies to benefit disabled people and to engage in "educational endeavors aimed at altering the beliefs and values of the nonhandicapped."[21]

Unlike many of her contemporaries in rehabilitation psychology, Dembo had hope for societal reforms and pushed psychologists to be more active in this process. Notably, however, her writing and speeches during the 1970s and early '80s did not emphasize the political and professional empowerment of disabled individuals themselves. She saw "nonhandicapped" people, like herself, as holding all of the decision-making power to change discriminatory policies and perceptions. Dembo held similarly paternalistic views about the potential impacts of disability self-advocacy as many other clinical professionals and rehabilitation specialists during this period.[22] Despite these doubts, many disability self-advocates were in fact actively and influentially engaged in pushing for change within the field of psychology and the wider world.

Self-Advocacy among Disabled Psychologists

As the disability self-advocacy movement became increasingly prominent in the late twentieth century, a new generation of disabled psychologists offered novel perspectives on disability discrimination and the potential for empowerment and social change. During this period, British and American self-advocates and scholars in sociology, social work, political science, and other fields established the "social model" of disability.[23] Some psychologists contributed to this scholarship and helped to promote these views of disability.

In the mid-1980s, Adrienne Asch was completing a PhD in social psychology at Columbia University. She was also a practicing clinical psychotherapist and an employment discrimination case investigator for New York State. Throughout her life, Asch—who was blind due to a medical intervention shortly after her birth—was an advocate for women and disabled people in many contexts, including as a bioethicist and disability scholar. In 1984, Asch contributed two articles on disability to a special issue of *American Psychologist*, APA's general interest professional journal. The first focused on disability as a civil rights issue in psychology and society and highlighted how laws and activism were shifting views on disability from individual and biological to interpersonal and political. Asch called on psychologists to embrace these trends by moving away from "exclusively clinical" research on disability and toward studies that engaged with the unique perspectives and experiences of disabled people. Instead of focusing on how *disabled people* impacted their families and nondisabled persons, she argued, psychologists should study how different *environmental contexts* affected disabled individuals.[24]

In a second article, Asch offered personal reflections on being a blind psychologist. She noted that disabled people from white, middle-class families, like herself, often thrived in educational settings as children, only to find that as adults they struggled to be accepted and to achieve rewarding employment that suited their capabilities. Describing her own experiences in professional contexts, she wrote, "I long for the day when I, other disabled psychologists, and other disabled people will go into any room in any convention, any meeting, or gathering, or job in the world and be greeted, evaluated, rejected, or accepted for who we are as total beings."

Asch also recalled an incident at a group-dynamics program she had attended, in which the participants were asked to stand under a sign representing their group identification. She had many options to choose from, but cognizant that she was the only disabled person in the room, Asch chose this sign. Another participant suggested that if Asch had selected "woman" over "disability," then she would have accused Asch of "denying." Asch retorted, "It's for people like you that I have to stand under that sign. You and your attitudes put me there, not my blindness itself."[25] Her decision to self-identify as having a disability, Asch emphasized, would not be needed in a more just world where blindness was inconsequential. In the present society though, Asch noted that disabled psychologists were forced to speak up about discrimination and organize their own professional forums to make it clear that they refused to be excluded.

Meanwhile, self-advocacy by disabled clinicians was influential within APA during the 1980s. One important focus group on disability issues was the Task Force on Psychology and the Handicapped, which had been created by the APA's Office on Social and Ethical Responsibility in 1979. The task force was established in part as a response to the US Rehabilitation Act of 1973, which made it unlawful for organizations receiving federal funding to discriminate against disabled people. Task force participants included multiple APA members with physical and sensory disabilities, as well as rehabilitation and clinical psychologists who specialized in disability research. Their primary focus was on removing barriers and providing supports for disabled psychologists related to professional training, conferences, and career goals.[26]

The task force referred to full participation of disabled practitioners in professional activities as a "civil rights issue" and argued that exclusion of psychologists based on their disability status "deprives society of the possible contributions of a significant number of its members, whose disabilities are extraneous to the positive contributions they might make." In 1984, the task force's final report called for APA to "educate psychologists and others regarding their own prejudices toward people with handicaps . . . [e]ncourage the study of people with disabilities from perspectives other than exclusively clinical," and ensure that disabled psychologists were "mainstreamed" in governance.[27] These were ambitious goals, which would require diffuse action and interventions over a long and ongoing period.

The final task force report recommended establishing a permanent APA committee to address ongoing issues and long-term goals. This would include developing strategies to reduce widespread employment discrimination against disabled psychologists and to encourage more nonclinical approaches to studying disability in the profession. The task force optimistically noted that efforts toward cultural change in psychology were underway and having an impact. As they put it, "Slowly we are starting to find ways to make nonhandicapped people want to change themselves, be concerned about others, and begin to value others who they previously devalued." In 1985, APA created a Committee on Disabilities and Handicaps. Its members included psychologists who conducted research in various areas, such as mental health, women's experiences with disability, spinal cord injuries, and rehabilitation psychology.[28]

Prominent rehabilitation psychologist Beatrice Wright was an early participant on the Committee on Disabilities and Handicaps. She had recently published a revision of her landmark textbook on disability, which took a much more psychosocial and environmental approach to rehabilitation compared to her original 1960 volume. In particular, Wright highlighted the "value-laden" beliefs and principles that guided her clinical work, including the fundamental rights of all disabled people, no matter how severe their disability. She noted, "We should be guided by *constructive views of life with a disability* in attempts to change attitudes positively" (emphasis in original). A persistent focus on presumed suffering and limits among disabled people did not promote such optimism.[29]

Wright did not identify as disabled, and in fact the APA Committee on Disabilities and Handicaps had very limited representation from disabled practitioners in its initial years. Nonetheless, many disabled psychologists believed that they had an important role to play in changing their colleagues' and clients' perceptions of disability. In 1979, the United States had just five deaf psychologists, including Irving King Jordan, who became deaf after a motorcycle accident at age 21. Several professors discouraged Jordan from pursuing a doctorate in clinical psychology. As he later recalled, "They said that deaf people simply didn't become clinical psychologists or succeed in clinical psychology programs. . . . Many people in the '60s, '70s, and even the '80s were counseled out of clinical psychology because they were deaf."[30]

Jordan followed through, becoming a professor at Gallaudet University a school committed to Deaf higher education (Deaf advocates preferentially use a capital *D* when describing Deaf culture and identity). In 1988, after student and faculty led protests demanding Deaf leadership, Jordan was named Gallaudet's first Deaf president. Soon thereafter, Gallaudet started a clinical psychology doctoral program, which succeeded in increasing the number of deaf people with PhDs in clinical psychology. However, the program's leaders struggled to find clinical internships and employment for their students—even in agencies that served primarily deaf people. No one ever questioned having hearing professionals work with deaf clients, but many were hesitant to allow deaf psychologists to see hearing *or* deaf patients.[31]

Throughout the late twentieth century, many disabled psychologists argued that they had much to offer patients, including unique viewpoints. In 1985, rehabilitation and clinical psychologist Carol Gill wrote about the importance of having "strong disabled role models" to inform and influence disabled individuals and their families. She noted research suggesting that disabled people may prefer, and benefit from, receiving care and support from disabled professionals. Gill experienced lasting effects from having polio as a child and used a motorized wheelchair. She proudly identified as a disabled person and lamented that nondisabled professionals played a dominant role in defining what research questions were pursued on disability. As a psychologist, Gill powerfully sought to combine her professional training and expertise with her own disability-related experiences, viewpoints, and ambitions.[32]

Asch similarly criticized the nature of existing disability research in psychology. Along with her social psychology colleague Michelle Fine, Asch wrote, "It is regrettable that people with disabilities, when studied or considered at all in most social-psychological literature, are examined only in ways that reinforce and perpetuate existing stereotypes rather than in ways that question and challenge them. To help provide an alternative model for engagement with disability, Fine and Asch published *Women with Disabilities: Essays in Psychology, Culture, and Politics* (1988). This edited volume highlighted the voices and experiences of disabled women and girls, and also offered psychological and political perspectives on their narratives.[33]

Professional Self-Advocacy and the Americans with Disabilities Act

During the 1980s, APA moved noticeably forward in acknowledging and addressing the concerns and challenges of disabled members. However, following the landmark passage of the Americans with Disabilities Act (ADA) in 1990, some disabled psychologists questioned how much progress was actually being achieved. APA had taken various steps to make its annual conventions more accessible.[34] Looking at the profession more broadly, though, clinical psychologist Alice L. Riger questioned APA's commitment to preventing discrimination against disabled people in psychology training programs and career advancement. In the early 1990s, Riger wrote letters to various APA officers and published a high-profile opinion piece criticizing ongoing professional inequities for disabled people and calling for clearer definitions, policies, and penalties addressing disability discrimination. Initially, she voiced her concerns to APA's Ethics Committee, asking whether they agreed with her view that training programs that were inaccessible to wheelchair users—like herself—were unethically prohibiting the inclusion of disabled people, and as a result should lose their APA accreditation.

In their response to Riger, the Ethics Committee stated that this was a legal not an ethical question. Such issues, they wrote, "involved decisions by groups of psychologists, and a member is only subject to investigation by the Ethics Committee based on individual responsibility."[35] Given APA's efforts in the 1970s and '80s to counteract its own institutional racism and sexism through the Board of Social and Ethical Responsibility for Psychology, it is remarkable that Riger's questions about structural injustices affecting disabled people in APA-accredited training programs were passed off as legal and not ethical concerns.[36] Clearly, APA was not interested in taking a larger, ethical stand about the full inclusion of disabled psychologists. The Committee's insistence that it only handled discrimination claims based on the actions of a single bad actor, but not organization-based decision-making, is also notable. This was a classic psychological response to disability issues—focusing on the thinking and actions of individuals rather than the impacts of social structures and environments. The Ethics Committee suggested that Riger should instead address her concerns to the APA Office of Accreditation.

In fact, Riger had already contacted the Accreditation Committee months earlier, and had voiced the position that the ethical question of disability inclusion was about more than APA's legal responsibilities under the ADA. She wrote, "Inaccessible programs have *always* breached our ethic of nondiscrimination, the ADA having no legal impact on this ethical principle, and therefore accrediting such programs has *always* been inappropriate" (emphasis in original). How long, she asked, would the Accreditation Committee continue to view it as acceptable for otherwise qualified disabled individuals to be excluded from some APA-accredited training programs?[37]

Riger raised similar concerns in an APA *Monitor* opinion piece, published in November 1992. She noted that career opportunities for psychologists with physical disabilities were limited by inaccessible workplaces, and suggested that nondisabled psychologists who continued to work in these locations without calling for change were also complicit, often without recognizing it.

Riger called for all psychologists to take a more active role in identifying and ending disability discrimination. She suggested,

> You can lobby your administration for improvements, insist on thoughtful, psychologically affirming environments, refuse to work in inaccessible spaces. . . . If you work in a medical setting, you can insist on devoting as much attention to the social, familial, and legal aspects of disability as to the biological. You can integrate people with disabilities into your social life, confront the managers of public establishments with access problems you notice and boycott offending establishments.[38]

For decades, psychologists had overlooked the potential for disabled people to successfully fight for their own inclusion and rights. In fact, Riger and other disabled psychologists *were* actively doing so—and *were trying* to convince their nondisabled colleagues to join them in these efforts.

Many of Riger's letters to APA officers were met with resistance and dismissal, but her efforts did contribute to momentum, which led to a new, although ultimately limited, APA Policy Statement on Full Participation for Psychologists with Disabilities, in 1997. The Committee on Disability Issues in Psychology composed an initial draft of the new policy a year earlier. After a preamble describing the exclusion of disabled psychologists from full participation in many APA activities, the draft stated, "Therefore be it resolved that APA will take reasonable steps to provide *full* access and participation in *all* activities, services, and resources of the association, to persons with disabilities" (emphasis added). Such policy statements passed through many levels of approval, concluding with the APA Council of Representatives. By the time this statement was published, having been approved by various APA bodies, its text and resolve had been watered down. It stated that APA would remain in "full compliance" with the ADA and pledged "to meet the reasonable requirements of its members with disabilities when providing the services and benefits to which all members are entitled."[39] A distinct shift in tone had taken place—from the principled demands of disability advocates into a much narrower, more legalistic statement.

In 1997, APA did take an important step forward by founding an Office on Disability Issues in Psychology, which was placed alongside the already existing APA offices on gender and racial diversity issues. Over the coming years, the Office on Disability Issues helped to organize various conferences and special journal issues on disability topics, pushed to expand coverage of disability issues in graduate training curricula, developed a mentoring program for disabled psychology graduate students, and sought to raise awareness about difficulties encountered by disabled practitioners. These efforts included the publication of various articles addressing the best practices and ADA-related responsibilities for psychology graduate programs and internship directors related to interviewing candidates and supporting disabled trainees.[40] During this period, APA took notice of some of the concerns and demands of disabled psychologists regarding the professional barriers that they faced. In the decades to come, psychologist self-advocates continued the push for change within APA and psychology broadly, calling for new perspectives on disability identity and reformed research approaches.

Promoting Inclusion, Diversity, and Pride

With the turn of the century on the horizon, many disabled psychologists and their allies began to adopt and promote more celebratory and empowered perspectives on the value of disability in their lives and professional careers. In 1997, Carol Gill wrote,

> We are beginning to oppose the sources of our disintegration as staunchly as we have fought environmental barriers and job discrimination. The emerging disability pride and culture movements many vanquish the most defeating and insidious form of oppression we have endured. Taught to disown our disabled parts and to avoid our disabled sisters and brothers, we have been profoundly handicapped in securing our rightful place in society.[41]

It was time, Gill and others argued, to tear down both the physical and psychological barriers that society—and the psychology profession—had erected, which discriminated against and stigmatized disabled people.[42] Gill made the case for the value of embracing a disability self-identity, forming a strong and vocal disability advocacy community, and achieving individual and societal empowerment through political activism and outward celebration of one's whole self, including their disability.

In the preface to her 1999 book, *What Psychotherapists Should Know about Disability*, clinical psychologist Rhoda Olkin described the evolution of her disability identity. Olkin had polio as an infant and as an adult continued to walk with a limp and used an electric scooter for daily mobility. She recounted the decades of her life during which she attempted to "pass" and distance herself from an outward presentation as a disabled person. Olkin identified a conference she attended, at which most of the participants were disabled professionals, as a turning point for her. The experience encouraged her to embrace a disability identity and helped her recognize that she could be a valuable role model for her disabled clients if she shared her own experiences.[43]

Over time, Olkin—like Gill and Asch—also began to reject some of the assumptions and methods underlying her own research. In 1999, she argued that much of the research currently being conducted on disability did more harm than good, and came to the conclusion that, "In place of a clarion call for more data I want to enter a plea for cessation of studies unless and until researchers approach the topic of disability from a different paradigm." Researchers, she noted, most often looked at the effects of individuals' disabilities on others rather than at how the social environment impacted disabled people. For instance, researchers rarely addressed how employer attitudes affected their decisions about whether to hire disabled job candidates.[44]

In a 2003 special issue of the *American Psychologist*, Gill and Olkin each encouraged psychologists to embrace "social model" perspectives as part of a "new paradigm" for conceptualizing and approaching disability. Gill and colleagues wrote, "Psychology's adoption of the new disability paradigm would further expand the discipline's focus on problems beyond the clinic to encompass social intervention, including issues of access, empowerment, and inclusion."[45] Along similar lines, Olkin and Pledger criticized the long-standing tendency among psychologists to relegate any interest in, or awareness of, disability issues to rehabilitation specialists and called for much broader exposure and engagement with disability across the psychology discipline.[46] Each set of authors criticized psychology's primary focus on individuals and called for more analysis of interactions between disabled people and their environments, as well as a shift toward facilitating greater empowerment rather than the continued pathologizing of disabled individuals.

Another important element of the new paradigm was assuring better opportunities and support for disabled psychology trainees and practitioners. As Gill put it, "For many psychologists, interns, and students with disabilities, the new paradigm validates their conviction that their productivity and competence are limited not by individual differences but by narrowly constructed standards and environmental obstacles."[47] These scholars' arguments had much in common with previous generations of disability advocates in psychology, who had promoted Lewinian perspectives and highlighted the minority group status of disabled people.

During the 1990s, Gill and Olkin benefited from the established status of the social model of disability and the new academic discipline of disability studies, as well as the recent passage of the ADA, to help bolster their positions. Nonetheless, they still faced an uphill battle among their colleagues in psychology. Few general training programs required coursework on disability issues and—although disabled people were identified in the APA Code of Ethics (2002) as a protected group—many disabled psychologists felt that their inclusion on this list was insufficiently backed by supportive and affirmative policies to combat discrimination.[48]

In 2019, a special issue of the *Journal of Social Issues* addressed the topic of "ableism" in psychology—a concept that situates disability discrimination in the same social framework as racism and sexism. This collection of articles was the third in a lineage of JSI special issues on disability, following in the footsteps of the 1948 effort organized by Lee Meyerson and another overseen by Fine and Asch in 1988. The 2019 editors acknowledged that "much work remains, and psychological research on disability as a social issue has not progressed as much as Fine and Asch had hoped."[49] Concrete achievements in the twenty-first century did not yet reflect the ambitions of the past, but efforts to change psychology's orientation toward disability continued.

Beginning in the 2010s, rehabilitation psychologist Erin E. Andrews contributed significantly to ongoing efforts aimed at integrating new narratives of disability into psychology training and practice, as well as enhancing the discipline's knowledge of the presence and status of its own disabled trainees and practitioners. Andrews had discovered disability scholarship and a new sense of community among disabled people as an undergraduate and was initially drawn to psychology after reading Olkin's work.[50] As part of her research, Andrews collected and analyzed data about disabled psychologists, with a focus on training experiences. She found that most of these psychologists had experienced disability discrimination as trainees, that few had disabled practitioners as mentors, and that many did not disclose their disability status or receive university services at all during their training, internship, and postdoctoral application process.

Andrews also drew upon APA data, collected from 2006 through 2012, which showed that 2 percent of psychology faculty, 3 percent of psychology doctoral students, and 1.4 percent of postdoctoral psychology interns identified as disabled under the ADA. Internship match rates were significantly lower for disabled students relative to other groups. Longer-term statistics also showed that, while the number of doctoral internships being completed by psychologists from racial minority groups had increased since the 1960s, the numbers for disabled psychologists had remained flat and had been eclipsed by the growing inclusion of other marginalized groups.[51] As self-advocates had previously suggested, advances in the acceptance and inclusion of minority groups in psychology were not being extended to disabled people. Importantly, Andrews noted, no data existed on disabled psychology trainees who were also members of racial minorities. The absence of this information prevented scholars from conducting important intersectional analyses of the demographic representation of disabled people—America's largest minority group—within the psychology profession.[52]

Andrews also helped formulate and promote a distinctive "diversity model" view of disability, which expanded upon the long-standing social model by viewing disabled people as a distinct cultural group due to their unique experiences. The social model had long been criticized, particularly by feminist scholars, for downplaying the relevance of impairment in people's lives—relative to societal sources of disability oppression. Liz Crow and other advocates had argued for a "reformed" social model, noting that some challenges of living with impairments would not simply go away if disability discrimination ended. By celebrating the valuable perspectives and experiences of life with (at times painful or disruptive) disabilities as a cultural phenomenon, the diversity model addressed some of the social model's shortcomings and encouraged empowerment through embracing a disability identity.[53] Andrews also promoted the identity-first construction "disabled person" as an expression of pride, while still noting the benefits of person-first language in combating the reduction of people to disabilities.

Expanding on Gill's work, Andrews and some of her disabled psychologist and rehabilitation colleagues also highlighted the importance of clinical practitioners as allies to disabled people. In a 2019 article, they encouraged rehabilitation specialists to "elicit discussions about disability with clients." For professional psychologists they noted, "Disability allyship involves critical self-reflection, attitude adjustment, and social action."[54] Pushing back on the traditional ambition of rehabilitation psychologists to direct their patients in coping with and overcoming disabilities, Andrews and colleagues identified a new role for clinicians in introducing and promoting the value of embracing a disability identity. Rehabilitation specialists could also assist their patients in recognizing solidarity with other disabled people, and in doing so encourage positive mindsets and empowerment. The authors suggested alternative methods for addressing a patient's disability identity, moving away from medical and functional terms and instead asking open-ended questions to begin a broad-based dialogue. For instance, "If there was a magic pill that would take away your disability, would you take it?" and "How do you define your disability identity or your connection to disability?" The resulting conversation would allow clinicians to gauge their patient's perspectives and goals, as well as provide opportunities to introduce the concept of disability as a valued form of diversity and unique cultural experience.[55]

Notably, proponents of the "new paradigm" and the "diversity model" also had their own blind spots. These psychologists rarely addressed intellectual and developmental disabilities or disabled children. Indeed, Olkin and Pledger dismissed the value of graduate psychology courses on intellectual disabilities for their tendency to "reflect the medical model of disability."[56] Further, Olkin and Pledger argued, "Psychology has generally viewed disability in the domain of rehabilitation psychology and this has conveyed that most psychologists do not need to be trained and skilled in working with people with disabilities and their families."[57] In fact, postwar psychologists in many specialty areas, including clinical, behaviorist, pediatric, developmental, and school psychology, frequently worked with disabled people and their families. Whereas, my survey of rehabilitation psychology's literature revealed that the field has had very little interest or engagement with intellectual, developmental, and childhood disabilities throughout its history.[58]

Over time, Andrews developed her own awareness of the "disability hierarchy," which favored people with physical disabilities over those with cognitive and other more stigmatizing conditions. Such interpretations were common in postwar clinical professions and bioethics, and even within disability advocacy communities.[59] By countering these views, Andrews hoped to encourage a more universal and collective disability identity. Her efforts included the Disabled Parenting Project—a central resource for support and engagement that welcomed and advocated on behalf of parents with all forms of disability, including intellectual. Part of the organization's work, she noted, involved countering the "internalized ableism" that some people with physical disabilities expressed regarding whether those with intellectual disabilities should be parents.[60]

Many, but certainly not all, postwar clinical psychologists who did primarily address intellectual disabilities maintained more pessimistic and pathological viewpoints. In the remainder of this chapter (as well as in chapter 4), I examine a parallel history of disability in psychology to the one described so far, and highlight a few psychologists who did push for more optimistic, accepting, and sociopolitical views of people with intellectual disabilities. There was very little awareness of, or engagement between, rehabilitation psychologists and intellectual disabilities specialists. Nonetheless, some prominent members of each group espoused similar views about the need for more positive, inclusive, and environmentally oriented perspectives on disability. They also faced similar forms of resistance from many of their colleagues in clinical psychology.

Normalization and Clinical Psychology

Postwar clinical psychologists who specialized in intellectual disabilities often trained and worked in residential institutions overseen by psychiatrist administrators. In these settings, clinical psychologists—who sometimes also had university appointments—conducted IQ testing, engaged in laboratory and clinical research involving residents, and designed and implemented educational, training, or disciplinary programs (chapter 4). As deinstitutionalization progressed during the 1970s and '80s, many clinical psychologists took positions in community-based clinics. Declining institutionalization was a direct threat to the careers of some clinical psychologists. Others were happy to move into new clinical settings but continued to be influenced—and in certain cases, appalled—by the conditions they had witnessed in institutions.

When Wolf Wolfensberger was training to be a clinical psychologist during the 1950s and '60s, he was shocked by the abuse and dehumanizing conditions in institutional settings. Wolfensberger later wrote that his anti-institutionalization sentiment began "in 1956 when my sense of justice was outraged by the conditions in the so-called 'back wards' of a mental institution in which I was then working as a clinical psychology trainee. The outrage was fueled in subsequent years by additional tours of, and episodes of work in, several other institutions of different kinds."[61] In 1957, Wolfensberger started his doctoral training in clinical psychology at the George Peabody College for Teachers in Nashville (now part of Vanderbilt University). At the time, it was the nation's only program that focused on mental retardation.[62]

As a PhD student, Wolfensberger's dismay grew while he worked summers as a staff psychologist at Muscatatuck State School for the Mentally Deficient in Butlerville, Indiana. This experience, he recalled, "bonded me to a commitment to mentally retarded people for the rest of my life."[63] Sociologists Harold Garfinkel and Erving Goffman—who wrote about total institutions, human degradation, and stigma in the 1950s and early 60s—also strongly shaped Wolfensberger, as did the anti-psychiatry sentiments of scholars like Thomas Szasz and R. D. Laing. These perspectives helped him to make sense of the staff and professional indifference and dehumanization that he encountered.[64]

In 1964, Wolfensberger became a mental retardation research scientist at the Nebraska Psychiatric Institute, with an academic appointment at the University of Nebraska Medical College. He arrived in Omaha at an opportune moment to push for major reforms. At this time, pediatrician Robert Kugel was serving as dean of the University of Nebraska Medical College. He was an early leader among pediatricians in promoting greater interest and engagement with the concerns and needs of children and families with mental retardation (chapter 2). Together, Kugel and Wolfensberger edited a landmark book, *Changing Patterns in Residential Services for the Mentally Retarded* (1969), which laid out an argument for, and approaches toward achieving, deinstitutionalization and enhanced community services for people with mental retardation. With spirited leadership from Wolfensberger and University of Nebraska Medical College psychiatrist Frank Menaloscino, Nebraska was one of the first US states to pass a comprehensive plan for deinstitutionalization, community inclusion, and support services for people with disabilities.[65]

During the early 1970s, Wolfensberger helped to popularize "normalization" in North America, drawing on the ideas and efforts of Scandinavian reformers Bengt Nirje and Karl Grunewald. As Wolfensberger described it in 1970, normalization meant helping "deviant" people to become "less deviant," without imposing social conformity on them. Becoming less deviant involved emphasizing similarities over differences from cultural norms, and valued personal traits rather than "negative" ones. In addition, normalization called for shaping the attitudes and values of society to be more accepting and tolerant of differences in people's appearance and behavior.[66] A central goal of normalization was to integrate institutionalized people back into society. Residential institutions, Wolfensberger argued, were not culturally normative places because they did not allow for typical social interactions, freedoms, and schedules. Thus, normalization could not be achieved when people lived in these locations.[67]

Wolfensberger further highlighted that, in addition to treating their patients as atypical persons, residential institutions were also frequently placed in socially devalued geographic locations—generally far from population centers or in rundown parts of town. This juxtaposition of institutional residents—along with the professionals who cared for them—with other socially marginalized places reiterated the message that these people were *less than* and existed apart from respected social destinations and activities.[68] In Nebraska and elsewhere, Wolfensberger sought to implement policies that normalized the daily lives, residential locations, and societal perceptions of people labeled with mental illness, retardation, and other disabilities. He also sought to make careers in mental retardation services more appealing and respected for future professionals. In Omaha, Wolfensberger instituted a summer internship program called Summer Work Experience and Training, or SWEAT, for high school and college students who might later specialize in disability services. The students actively engaged with and learned from disabled people, getting to know them on a more personal basis. Over the course of his career, Wolfensberger hoped to encourage greater acceptance and inclusion of disabled people in society through such "life-sharing" activities and communities. He and Menolascino were particularly inspired by Jean Vanier's L'Arche, in which people chose to incorporate their lives for a time into a small community of disabled and nondisabled people.[69]

Over the first decade of his career, Wolfensberger moved away from his initial identity as a clinical psychologist. By 1970, he had reason to believe that his views were becoming too controversial for academic clinical professionals, thus necessitating his move to the School of Education at Syracuse University. As Wolfensberger later put it, "Unlike other professors who perished when they did not publish, I perished in good part because of *what* I published" (emphasis in original).[70] Indeed, he had helped to foment a movement that many clinicians were not yet ready to accept. Wolfensberger argued that residential institutions reflected society's indifference to, and rejection of, people with mental retardation and other disabilities. These institutions, he strongly believed, were not therapeutic locations but stigmatizing ones, and they needed to be fully depopulated because, by their very nature and function, they could not be reformed or improved.

Resistance to Deinstitutionalization in Clinical Psychology

During the 1970s, normalization was a touchstone concept in the deinstitutionalization movement. While it was the inspiration and basis for significant change, a common ambition of many normalization advocates—the complete deinstitutionalization of people with intellectual and developmental disabilities—was the target of significant criticism and pushback. Depopulating institutions was only an initial step, and often the easiest and most cost effective one, in the process of achieving normalization and societal inclusion. Comprehensive community support and full integration required the creation of new types of housing and a network of services, as well as changing people's willingness to accept more diverse neighbors. As scholars and reformers have since noted, these goals were often only partially or fleetingly realized.[71]

Many clinical psychologists and administrators of residential institutions criticized normalization as an unproven and potentially harmful ideal, which was valued-laden rather than based on empirical scientific evidence. As part of this, they questioned whether the policy of complete deinstitutionalization was the best option for all people with intellectual disabilities. One prominent critic of complete deinstitutionalization among clinical psychologists was Edward Zigler. Like Wolfensberger, Zigler trained in clinical psychology during the 1950s and had significant experience working in residential institutions for people with intellectual disabilities. Zigler joined the Yale Department of Psychology in 1959. At Yale, Zigler moved away from the mainstream of clinical psychology and established himself in the burgeoning academic field of developmental psychology as a specialist in mental retardation. Zigler went on to receive tenure at Yale and never left—aside from the time he spent directing the US Office of Child Development and US Children's Bureau. Along with pediatrician Robert Cooke and Lyndon Johnson advisor Sargent Shriver (chapter 2), Zigler also helped to develop and lead the US government's Head Start program for early childhood education, which began in 1965.[72]

Zigler's research focused on children's responses to the social deprivation of residential institutions, as well as certain community settings, and how these environments affected a child's desire for attention and their performance on tasks—like IQ tests. He was a strong proponent of the "developmental perspective" on intellectual disabilities, which held that most affected individuals developed in the same ways as "normal" children but at a slower pace and with lower overall achievement. Zigler also believed that some children were organically different and thus did not follow the normal course of intellectual development. This distinction, which he called the "two-group approach," suggested that many children with IQs above 50 developed atypically because of environmental or complex genetic causes. Meanwhile, Zigler held that others, especially children with a lower IQ, were affected by a discrete, pathological difference.[73]

Among postwar clinical psychologists, Zigler's extensive investment in designing and implementing social policy through government agencies was quite unusual. However, when it came to his clinically based, empirical, and individual-focused research methods, Zigler retained a much more mainstream orientation. While Zigler was sympathetic to many of the goals of normalization, he was also a critic of psychologists who promoted its implementation based on value-laden arguments rather than hard-nosed scientific evidence. In 1976 testimony before Congress, Zigler referred dismissively to normalization as "a banner in search of some data."[74]

Zigler was unmoved by what he called the "social address" arguments of Wolfensberger and other normalization proponents, who held that residential institutions were unavoidably stigmatizing and harmful because of their atypical environments and location in socially devalued and isolated places. He and his coauthors believed that the specific internal environment of each institution needed to be studied to determine its distinctive value and efficacy for certain individuals.[75] In line with other professionals who resisted calls for complete deinstitutionalization, Zigler and his coauthors argued that there were good institutions and bad ones, and that children experienced social deprivation in community settings as well. Zigler and his coauthors maintained that institutions were not inherently pathological, even though they believed that some people were. In his view, institutions could be reformed and improved. Most important for success was the proper matching of individual people to specific residential settings, which might be large or small, isolated or community-based, highly restrictive or more open and loosely regulated.[76]

During the 1980s, tensions over normalization and deinstitutionaliza-tion were high among clinical psychologists who specialized in intellectual disabilities. Some psychologists were dependent on the continued existence of residential institutions to maintain their research agendas—or even their careers. Others were more directly concerned about the degree to which the ideals of normalization were driving social policy toward deinstitutional-ization in the absence of robust empirical evidence. At the same time, many advocates who drew on value-laden arguments for immediate and complete deinstitutionalization were no longer willing to wait for psychological sci-entists to continue turning institutionalized people's lives into another con-trolled experiment.

In 1989, clinical psychologists Stephen Greenspan and Mary Cerreto noted the ways in which debates over normalization had come to reflect broader divides in the psychology discipline between experimental scientists and clinical reformers, like themselves. As they put it, "[while others] lament the lack of empirical validation for normalization, we accept it, because value systems cannot, and should not, be subjected to empirical testing."[77] Zigler and those who called for more empirical scientific validation retorted that psychologists who supported normalization were willing to suppress find-ings that challenged their belief in the benefits of complete deinstitutional-ization rather than interrogating the implications of such findings.[78]

Wolfensberger, for one, was strongly committed to empirically assessing the achievement and impacts of normalization through the development and application of his PASS (Program Analysis of Service Systems) rating tool. Indeed, while Zigler was primarily concerned with the responses of individuals to certain environments, Wolfensberger focused on measuring the degree of normalization and community inclusion achieved by specific service environments for people with intellectual disabilities. Wolfensberger certainly appreciated the importance of backing social policy with the "data" that Zigler and others demanded, but he also believed that the most impor-tant issues "have not been, are not now, and never will be decided on the basis of 'research,' or even on the basis of empiricism and evidence. They will be settled on the plane of values and ideologies."[79] As Zigler positioned himself on what he called the "science side" of the normalization issue, Wolfensberger pointed out that scientific research was not itself immune to the influences of ideologies, even if many psychologists failed or refused to admit this reality.[80]

Similar debates about the relative importance and legitimacy of scientific methods versus other value-laden beliefs and approaches were widespread in late twentieth-century clinical psychology. I expand on this history in chapter 4. As is already becoming clear, defensiveness about the unique validity and power of empirical, experimentally controlled, and individual-focused methods for generating knowledge related to disability assessment and interventions often came in conflict with efforts to promote more positive, inclusive, and sociopolitical views.

Positive Psychology and Intellectual Disabilities

By the mid-1990s, tensions began to settle down among clinical psychologists in the normalization debate. Deinstitutionalization had run its course, closing some of the most controversial residential institutions—like Willowbrook State School in New York City—and leaving many others with significantly reduced populations, primarily older people or those with more "severe" disabilities. Amid the ongoing Human Genome Project, greater interest in the genetic causes of intellectual disabilities also emerged in clinical psychology. In 1995, Elisabeth Dykens made the case that psychologists should do more to study forms of intellectual disability that were linked to discrete genetic causes. The "new genetics," she argued, presented psychologists with new opportunities to examine specific "behavioral phenotypes," which were present in rare genetic conditions such as Prader-Willi, fragile X, and Williams syndromes.[81]

Focusing on one or a few rare genetic conditions led some psychologists, including Dykens, to develop closer and more holistic relationships with her patients and their families. I have observed a similar trend among other clinical professionals who focused on genetic conditions (chapter 5).[82] During the mid-2000s, Dykens began to embrace and integrate thinking from the fledgling area of "positive psychology" into her research and practice. Martin Seligman initially popularized positive psychology when he was APA president in the late 1990s. This specialty area and orientation privileged beneficial individual traits and strengths, with a goal of helping people to achieve the "good life."[83] Seligman directly influenced Dykens through an online course. Eventually, she noted to him that positive psychology had not addressed disability.

In the early 2000s, clinical psychologists had begun to more actively identify both the strengths and weaknesses of their patients (chapter 4).

Soon thereafter, Dykens highlighted that no theoretical framework yet existed in the area of intellectual and developmental disabilities for engaging with personal strengths, but that positive psychology appeared to offer a model.[84] In 2006, she wrote, "While mental retardation is indeed defined by negatives, and the field caught up with the external, I propose a future research and practice agenda based on *positive internal* states, including happiness, contentment, hope, engagement, and strengths" (emphasis in original).[85] In line with disability self-advocates in psychology, Dykens promoted moving away from a focus on negatives and deficits in intellectual disabilities and toward researching positives and strengths.

Some psychologists who focused on specific genetic conditions involving intellectual disabilities had begun pointing out common "core strengths" in these populations. For instance, Down syndrome was often associated with a happy and sweet personality; people with Prader-Willi syndrome were frequently good at puzzles; and individuals with Williams syndrome could be very musically talented. Dykens and her colleagues recognized that these were stereotypes, which did not universally apply to all individuals with these conditions. Nonetheless, they suggested that recognition and promotion of these traits among clinicians might offer new chances to facilitate enhanced individual happiness, engagement, and enjoyment of activities.[86]

Still, while positive psychology emphasized a more optimistic and affirmative view of life with disabilities, the field primarily did so by continuing to focus on an individual's internal contentment rather than on social oppression, empowerment, identity, and reform. Seligman had initially intended positive psychology to also focus on bringing about more positive social institutions, but little research was ever done with this ambition in mind. Given postwar clinical psychologists' tendency to focus on individuals, this is not a surprising outcome. The field of positive psychology instead moved toward highlighting individual resiliency to adversity.[87]

Relative to decades of pessimism and ongoing psychological research on the apparent deficits of, and harms purportedly caused by, disabled people, the fact that positive psychologists actually accepted that disabled people *did have* positive traits and experiences worth studying could be considered a major step forward. However, the dominance of individual-based thinking remained infused within this new approach. Indeed, when it came to disability, positive psychology was still representative of the largely asocial and apolitical orientation of its parent discipline.

Conclusions

Many postwar clinical psychologists contributed to the development and promotion of more optimistic, accepting, and sociopolitical views of people with disabilities. Importantly, this included numerous disability self-advocates who worked from within the profession to bring about positive change. The approaches of self-advocates evolved over the postwar period, from a minority group framing in the 1950s and '60s, to civil rights-based arguments, and eventually to new paradigms promoting social empowerment, diversity, and the celebration of a disability identity. Defying the expectations of some professionals, disability self-advocates in psychology took on a leading role in making change happen and recruited their colleagues to join the fight.

Along the way, a few common threads of resistance to new perspectives and approaches to studying and supporting disabled people regularly appeared. First, most psychologists remained focused on addressing individual disabled patients—by characterizing specific deficits, identifying anticipated or actual strengths, and defining what type of environment was most conducive to an individual's success. As part of this, psychological research highlighted the presumed negative impacts of disabled individuals on their families and society instead of considering the effects of discrimination by the nondisabled majority, highlighting structural oppression, and incorporating the perspectives and experiences of disabled people. The individual-level orientation of psychologists extended to their perceptions of accountability for disability discrimination. In the 1990s, APA's Committee on Ethics addressed shortcomings in accommodating or respecting disabled psychologists in terms of the failings of individual bad actors rather than structural factors—like inaccessible training programs and workplaces.

Second, clinical psychologists resisted calls to view and address disability discrimination in the same ways as they did racial and gender disparities. While psychologists made influential arguments about the appropriateness of social and school integration by race and the need for greater racial and gender diversity in their discipline, when it came to full deinstitutionalization of disabled people, many were hesitant and demanded more evidence. Even psychologists who focused on social reform did not view disability discrimination as an interesting or important issue that was on par with societal oppression by race and gender. Disabled psychologists argued that APA

also did not show the same vigor or moral leadership in welcoming and supporting the full inclusion of disabled trainees and practitioners as it had in
increasing the discipline's commitment to gender and racial diversity. (Notably, even with these efforts, the racial diversity of psychologists in the
2010s remained well below representative.)[88]

Third, clinical psychologists almost always approached intellectual disabilities as a separate category from physical disabilities. Rehabilitation
psychologist Beatrice Wright's concept of "spread"—the tendency for negative reactions to one personal trait, such as a physical disability, to lead to
the presumption of other negative individual attributes, like an intellectual
disability—offers one potential explanation for this pattern. Awareness and
internalization of a "disability hierarchy," which placed people with physical
disabilities above those with cognitive and other more stigmatizing conditions, may account for rehabilitation specialists' and self-advocates' tendency
to avoid association with, or engagement in advocacy related to, people with
intellectual disabilities.[89] A sense of shared experiences, disability identity,
or minority group status among these populations was absent from the
discourse of postwar clinical psychology and psychologist self-advocates.
Whatever the impetus, separating out professional specialization and social
activism for physical disabilities from intellectual disabilities undercut the
potential for more collaborative and uniform sociopolitical viewpoints and
efforts.

My analysis of psychologists' promotion of, and resistance to, more positive, inclusive, and sociopolitical views of disability continues in chapter 4.
Meanwhile, in the next chapter, I turn to the history of pediatrics. Somewhat
surprisingly, pediatricians were less actively involved in caring for children
with intellectual and developmental disabilities during the mid-twentieth
century in comparison to clinical psychologists who specialized in this area.
Pediatricians began to develop a greater interest in children with intellectual
and developmental disabilities during the 1960s, and spent decades trying
to catch up with other professional fields—including psychiatry, education,
and social work—to take on a more recognized leadership role in the area
of developmental disabilities. In pediatrics, this transition was powerfully
driven by practitioners who were themselves parents of disabled individuals.
They advocated for views other than pessimism and stigma, as well as for
enhancing the prestige of research and services in this area.

2

Pediatrics

Moves toward Leadership in

Developmental Disabilities

In 2007, reflecting on her six-decade career in medicine, pediatrician Margaret Giannini identified a key moment, around 1950, when the trajectory of her life's work began to change. She recalled,

> There were five sets of parents who had children with intellectual disabilities— we said then retarded—who went to every teaching hospital in New York to plead for a clinic to which they could bring their children when they were sick. Not for their disability, but just when they were sick, if they had a cough or if they had a temperature . . . but doctors would not see these children.

Giannini was shocked to learn that other pediatricians were refusing to care for disabled children and also recommending institutionalization to their parents as the only option to avoid ruinous effects for their family's well-being and social status. She was "emotionally taken" by the parents' struggles and soon agreed to see children with mental retardation one morning a week at New York Medical College, in Manhattan, where she was on the faculty.[1]

A single morning each week quickly grew to two, and then four. Soon, Giannini decided to fully commit and requested space to open a mental retardation clinic at New York Medical College. Her dean supported the plan and granted her an out-of-the-way space in the basement near a boiler room, which had a separate entrance. She noted, "The faculty complained because they didn't want these kids. . . . They didn't want to see them. The other patients were kind of annoyed. So we were in the basement." Giannini recognized right away that she did not have adequate knowledge to help all of her patients, so she found volunteers from other disciplines who contributed their expertise. Then she got to fundraising. A decade later, when the US government began catching up in recognizing the unmet needs of children and families with mental retardation, her clinic was well positioned to compete for funding. Federal money was used to help build a much larger and more attractive space for the Mental Retardation Institute.[2]

Giannini went on to become president of the American Association on Mental Deficiency, a member of the American Academy of Pediatrics' (AAP) Committee on Children with Handicaps, and the first director of the National Institute of Handicapped Research. She was one of the earliest postwar pediatricians to openly push past the discouragement and disinterest of her colleagues and help fill the long-standing pediatrics leadership gap in the area of developmental disabilities. Giannini's exposure to the great needs of children and families was the impetus for her initial investment in mental retardation. However, her long-term success in the area also depended on new opportunities for professional support and career advancement, facilitated by the growing interest of professional organizations, influential families, and the US government in better supporting children with developmental disabilities. Indeed, as I explore in this chapter, pediatricians' transition toward greater engagement in training, research, and services related to developmental disabilities was often a matter of both passion *and* prestige.

Postwar pediatricians followed various pathways toward increased involvement with, and specialized interest in, children and families with developmental disabilities. For some, a surprise encounter with disability—in their patients, their own children, or the wider community—was a defining moment, when they suddenly realized how poorly prepared and ill-informed they were about how to respond and help. A few of these pediatricians went on to push for improvements in medical school training, residency programs, and continuing education, which would expose physicians to the various challenges, strengths, and resource needs of disabled people. As part of this, promoters of increased pediatrics involvement in developmental disabilities recognized that waiting for physicians to organically develop a passion for working with this population—like Giannini had—would not be sufficient to address the area's already significant workforce needs. Instead, they looked to bring more opportunities and greater professional status to research, training, and the clinical care involving children with developmental disabilities.

When Giannini created her clinic in 1950, she found no existing model of a small, outpatient mental retardation specialty center. Indeed, the appropriate role for pediatricians in caring for children and families with mental retardation, beyond their initial diagnosis, was not yet defined. Giannini cobbled together a team of specialist consultants in medicine and other clinical fields and took on the role of director.[3] As similar clinics opened over the next two decades, other pediatricians also sought to claim the most prestigious leadership positions as team leaders and care-coordinators for patients and families with mental retardation.[4] In the broader area of pediatric rehabilitation, AAP's Committee on the Handicapped Child promoted the view in 1956 that "a pediatrician is best suited for this role [medical director] since by virtue of his training and temperament he can fulfill the demands of the child and parents, and understand the drives of professional workers. His knowledge of growth and development gives the pediatrician a high priority for the role of team leader." The AAP report also diminished psychiatrists' appropriate roles, characterizing them as collaborators but not team leaders.[5]

During the late 1950s, as more societal and medical attention was given to mental retardation, pediatricians found that there were plenty of affected children and families in their communities who were in need of clinical care and support. However, psychiatrist administrators of residential institutions often held the primary professional jurisdiction and government backing for overseeing this population. Even as postwar pediatricians promoted an identity as uniquely qualified team leaders, they found that to take on these new roles in developmental disabilities, more state governments would have to recognize their expertise in the area. This meant wrestling professional jurisdiction away from psychiatrists, who pediatricians argued—with reasonable accuracy—were not all that interested in children with mental retardation.[6]

As part of their efforts, pediatricians encouraged a shift in training, research, and care for mental retardation away from isolated residential institutions and to community locations—like universities, outpatient clinics, and private practices—where they had more influence. Although many pediatricians in the early 1960s still viewed institutions as an option that needed to be available, they opposed institutionalization before age six, suggesting that preschool children—notably a demographic that more regularly visited their offices—were best raised at home.[7]

As deinstitutionalization progressed in the 1970s, clinical psychologists were increasingly hired to be members of pediatrician-led, community-based clinical care teams for children with developmental disabilities. While the two fields occasionally collaborated on research, their professional roles were generally quite distinct in these settings. Pediatricians were most often involved in the initial diagnosis, care-coordination, and community-based advocacy, whereas clinical psychologists' primary roles included IQ testing, developing and implementing educational programs, and research. As physicians, pediatricians held significantly more clinical and community prestige than PhD-holding psychologists, so pediatricians rarely viewed clinical psychologists as direct competitors in establishing their leadership in developmental disabilities.

This chapter explores the evolving participation of pediatricians in caring and advocating for children and families with developmental disabilities throughout the postwar period. During the 1960s and '70s, this area was transformed from a professional backwater into a more active and highly regarded specialty of pediatric research, training, and practice. These changes were strongly influenced by parent advocates—some of who were physicians themselves—who in the decades immediately following World War II increasingly organized to demand better resources, opportunities, and inclusion for their disabled children.[8] Postwar pediatricians were undoubtedly influenced by parent activism and other sociopolitical efforts to promote greater inclusion for disabled people. However, other professional factors played major roles as well. In this chapter, I ague that many pediatricians' choices to pursue more knowledge, specialization, and engagement in developmental disabilities were also motivated by new career pathways and markers of prestige, which rewarded investments in training, services, and research in this area.

At the same time, the long-term and time-intensive nature of comprehensively supporting children and families with developmental disabilities conflicted with the many professional and financial benefits of focusing on acute conditions, for which there existed successful—and easily billable—curative interventions. While the hope for new cures and preventative measures drew many pediatricians to disability-related research, others viewed the reality that most children with developmental disabilities would never "get better" as a major disincentive to being involved. Ultimately, a combination of both new professional optimism *and* career opportunities played a significant part in making pediatricians' work in developmental disabilities what it is today—a more appealing but still quite difficult and poorly compensated area of expertise and practice.

Recruiting Pediatricians to Mental Retardation

In 1953, prominent Yale pediatrician Grover Powers was the second annual recipient of the American Pediatric Society's most prestigious award, the John Howland Medal, recognizing lifetime achievement in pediatric professional leadership. Powers used the occasion as an opportunity to address the issue of pediatric practice, research, and education in mental retardation. He began, "I offer no apology for my subject. Here are major problems perhaps as old as human life itself but still too low on the totem poles of medical respectability and of scientific concern."[9] Parent advocates, Powers noted, were "way out in front" of professionals in providing guidance and support to families of children with mental retardation and had been playing an important role in "raising the sights" of many clinical and educational personnel.

Powers was one of these parents' most important recruits. He had recently been named the first chair of the National Association for Retarded Children's (NARC) Scientific Research Advisory Board.[10] As the long-standing chair of the Department of Pediatrics at Yale School of Medicine, Powers had overseen, since 1941, clinical rotations that brought medical students, interns, residents, and fellows to the Southbury Training School—a residential institution in rural Connecticut—for training, service, and research experience in mental retardation.[11] In his Howland Award address, Powers promoted this training model, which involved direct and sustained academic links between Yale and Southbury Training School. He noted, "Affiliation of training schools with university departments of medicine, psychology, psychiatry, social science, and education enhances the prestige and morale of training school personnel—something which should not be needed but definitely is at this time." These opportunities helped Yale and Southbury to attract highly regarded young physicians to research and service in mental retardation—an area of medicine, he suggested, that many assumed could only attract clinicians "with second rate abilities."[12] At Yale and Southbury, Powers trained some of the towering figures of the next generation, including Robert Cooke, who became pediatrician-in-chief at Johns Hopkins School of Medicine and one of medicine's most prominent advocates for children with developmental disabilities.

NARC also had significant success in attracting major figures in pediatrics and other specialties to their Scientific Research Advisory Board during the 1950s, who helped the association influence AAP and in particular its Committee on the Handicapped Child. Some NARC parent advocates were highly critical of many physicians' encouragement of residential institutionalization for children with mental retardation from a very young age.[13] In 1956, the Committee on the Handicapped Child came out strongly against this practice and expressed unanimous agreement that "mentally retarded and crippled children should continue to live in their own homes and receive training and care in that environment and that of their community, as long as it is feasible and practical to keep them here."[14] Even among pediatricians with more progressive views on the issue of institutionalization for mental retardation though, there remained a general assumption that many more "severely" affected children would eventually require an institutional placement, at least for a time. Some noted that preschool-age children reared in supportive family homes were "more easily adjusted and . . . taught" when they did enter residential settings later in childhood.[15] During the 1950s, the Committee on the Handicapped Child contributed to surveying and improving the conditions of residential institutions and also actively encouraged better knowledge and training for physicians on childhood disabilities.[16]

Other prominent pediatricians developed an interest in developmental disabilities due to additional influences. Paul W. Beaven, a former AAP president, became concerned about children with mental retardation through his long-standing work with adoption agencies. Over the decades of his career, Beaven's views evolved significantly. He recounted, "In common with most physicians, I used to advise all parents with retarded children to put them out of the home as soon as the diagnosis was made. Most often this was made at birth or soon afterward."[17] The goal was to prevent parental attachment, which would make decisions more difficult when—inevitably, physicians presumed—institutionalization became necessary later in childhood. Beaven grew to believe that "mildly or moderately retarded children" should remain in their parents' homes throughout childhood or be eligible for adoption—instead of immediate institutionalization—because, he had learned, there were families willing to raise them.[18]

In 1958, Beaven and multiple other AAP members sent letters to the Academy's executive board arguing for a new committee specific to mental retardation.[19] The board passed this suggestion along to the Committee on the Handicapped Child, which was "vigorous and unanimous in its insistence" that mental retardation should remain an integral part of their work. The Committee strongly opposed any moves to separate out mental retardation from other forms of childhood disability but also recognized the need to work closely on this issue with the newly established AAP Section on Child Development. Further discussion led to the formation of a section subcommittee on mental retardation, chaired by pediatrician Robert Kugel, director of the Child Development Clinic at the University of Iowa.[20] Other members included pediatricians Hulda Thelander and Hilda Knobloch, who were also early leaders in providing clinical services for and training related to children with developmental disabilities. Kugel was dismissive of the need for a separate committee on mental retardation, noting "there is a certain vocal group in pediatrics, interested in mental retardation, who are looking for some 'place in the sun.' "[21] As research and services related to mental retardation became more prestigious and lucrative around 1960, influential pediatrics groups increasingly sought to control the area rather than to avoid it.

Harry Waisman, a pediatrician at the University of Wisconsin who also held a PhD in biochemistry, was another major proponent of greater AAP involvement in mental retardation.[22] In the late 1950s, he was engaged in research on the effects of phenylpyruvate buildup in rats, which in humans brought about the condition phenylketonuria (PKU), a well-known cause of mental retardation that could be prevented using severe dietary restrictions.[23] Though quite rare, PKU offered an inspiring model of hope for finding and preventing discrete causes of mental retardation. Waisman pushed for greater AAP investment in mental retardation from the camp of basic researchers, who were not well represented within the Academy, but held great prestige and generated valuable optimism among their colleagues that new treatments were possible. In 1961, Waisman contacted Kugel to suggest that a special conference session on PKU research would be an appropriate next step for the Academy to further its efforts on mental retardation.[24]

Around 1960, significant new sources of financial support for basic research on mental retardation emerged. NARC funded a wide range of basic research in many disciplines and was particularly enthusiastic about supporting advances in PKU prevention, including universal newborn screening programs.[25] Another major benefactor to mental retardation research, beginning in the late 1950s, was the Joseph P. Kennedy Jr. Foundation, overseen by Robert Sargent and Eunice Kennedy Shriver. Eunice was the sister of John, Robert, and Ted Kennedy, and of Rosemary Kennedy, who had been diagnosed as "mentally retarded." Following the catastrophic effects of a lobotomy, Rosemary was institutionalized in 1941. During the late 1950s, and certainly with the experiences of their sister in mind, the Kennedy Foundation began distributing significant funding to support research related to mental retardation.[26]

Waisman was a major recipient of Kennedy Foundation funding for his work on PKU. Another was Cooke, who developed a strong relationship with the Shrivers and soon received a $1.275 million grant to fund mental retardation research at Johns Hopkins in many clinical and basic science fields. Cooke had convinced the Shrivers that mental retardation required a multidisciplinary approach. They requested that he be designated as director of the mental retardation research program at Johns Hopkins, putting him in charge of distributing much of the funding.[27] Around the same time, Cooke was also named to the Grover F. Powers Professorship, a new and prestigious position funded by NARC. In this position Cooke was called upon "to develop a climate in which the attention of young scientists will be attracted to the possibilities offered by research on mental retardation." With scientists in short supply, Cooke noted, unique funding efforts were necessary to attract investigators to an area that many assumed to be unrewarding.[28]

Cooke also had a personal connection to NARC and the Shrivers because he had two young daughters with significant developmental disabilities. Robyn and Wendy were born in 1948 and 1951, respectively, when Cooke was still at Yale. They lived at home for most of their young lives before being placed in the Southbury Training School as teenagers. In the mid-1960s, both sisters were diagnosed with cri du chat syndrome, a rare chromosomal disorder recently delineated by Jérôme Lejeune in France, who had also helped to identify the link between Down syndrome and trisomy 21. Robyn died in 1967, shortly after moving to Southbury. Wendy lived into her mid-fifties and was probably the oldest person alive with cri du chat for much of her life.[29]

Cooke's family experiences undoubtedly influenced his interest and commitment to improved research and training in mental retardation. Professionally, he was also in the right place at the right time for significant career advancement in the area. Writing to the Shrivers after they visited Johns

Hopkins in 1959, Cooke described his investment in mental retardation, stating, "I can only reiterate a rather considerable interest based on personal problems as well as a rather long history of professional association with institutional, hospital, and clinical facilities for mentally retarded children."[30] Cooke and the Shrivers shared significant common interests and experiences—and with Eunice's brother running for president, their work had just begun.

Enhanced Federal Support

The election of John F. Kennedy in 1960 was a watershed moment for societal investment in research, training, and clinical services in developmental disabilities. Kennedy was committed to improving child health generally. Cooke and the Shrivers worked together to ensure that major new funding for mental retardation was also part of the conversation. One important Administration effort sought to expand the National Institutes of Health's (NIH) support for pediatric research and clinical services through the creation of a new institute. Cooke was centrally involved in the planning and promotion for an institute on child health and development, which he hoped would fund more mental retardation research programs like the one that he developed and led at Johns Hopkins with support from the Kennedy Foundation.[31]

In 1961, Cooke was also a participant on the President's Panel on Mental Retardation. The panel comprised 26 members with diverse backgrounds, including physicians, basic scientists, educators, lawyers, and a parent representative from NARC. Cooke later commented that this mixture of interest groups was groundbreaking and important but also brought to the surface various tensions. The laboratory scientists, including Nobel laureate geneticist Joshua Lederberg, felt that more basic research was the best approach to mental retardation. Whereas, educators on the panel resisted the view that mental retardation was primarily a medical problem. These debates intersected with ongoing discussions in Congress about funding a new institute on child health and human development. Some educators and basic researchers on the panel resisted the clinicians' desire to bolster support for a new institute in their final report.[32] Differing views on the nature of mental retardation, and what to do about it, cropped up throughout the panel's discussions and remained major areas of disagreement among professionals for decades to come.

Eunice Shriver sat in on meetings of the President's Panel on Mental Retardation as a consultant. She was instrumental in organizing its creation but quite disappointed with its initial draft report because for her it did not appear to suggest anything new and different. Shriver expressed these misgivings to her brother, the president. As Cooke recalled, he was playing tennis with the Shrivers one day at their estate in Virginia when John Kennedy called asking for some novel ideas for his upcoming address on mental health and mental retardation. Cooke immediately went inside and drafted a proposal for funding university-affiliated clinical facilities (UAF), which he envisioned as centers for multidisciplinary training in mental retardation. President Kennedy ended up promoting this model in his address. Funding to construct UAFs was ultimately included in the Mental Retardation and Community Mental Health Centers Construction Act of 1963 (PL 88-164). Its passage came a year after Congress also approved the creation of the National Institute of Child Health and Human Development (NICHD).

In his speeches to various medical and disability advocacy audiences during the early 1960s, Cooke presented NICHD as pursuing a distinct approach from much of medicine, which focused on preventing and curing acute and deadly diseases. The new Institute's research would instead encourage a more longitudinal orientation on normal and atypical aspects of human development. Cooke also offered recommendations for how medical students could be more adequately trained in the area of mental retardation. He suggested that they should be assigned to a specific patient with a severe handicapping condition early in medical school, so that students could participate in care and planning with them and their families over an extended period. In the process, he argued, students would learn about community resources for disabled people and the other professions involved in care and support. As he put it, perhaps reflecting on his own family experiences, "Nothing, yes nothing, is as maturing as personal involvement with a family confronted with a seriously handicapped infant or child."[33] Cooke's idea was radical—he sought to greatly enhance medical students' awareness and empathy for disability experiences. Indeed, the wide-scale adoption of such an approach in the 2020s would still be quite revolutionary.

President Kennedy signed PL 88-164 just a few weeks before he was assassinated. Cooke had heavily influenced its contents. Title I invested in the construction of physical buildings for mental retardation and human development–focused research centers, as well as clinical facilities for mental retardation training and services, which would be affiliated with universities. These facilities were initially called Mental Retardation Research Centers (MRRC) and UAFs. Later, they became known as Eunice Kennedy Shriver Intellectual and Developmental Disabilities Research Centers and University Centers of Excellence in Developmental Disabilities. In promoting these investments, Cooke had noted that, before 1963, almost no federal or state funding existed for mental retardation services and training at universities or within communities. Rather, most training in mental retardation for clinical professions took place "in the depressing atmosphere of large, state-supported, many-purpose residential institutions where the medical and social failures of the community are concentrated."[34] With the newly funded centers, medical students, residents, and fellows could be trained in university hospital–based in-patient units for mental retardation and would follow their patients as they were integrated and supported within their local communities. Training in mental retardation was moving to more appealing, optimistic, and research-oriented locations, which Cooke believed would encourage greater medical interest, investment, and prestige.

As UAFs were developed across the country during the 1960s and '70s, they implemented a multidisciplinary training and team approach to clinical services in mental retardation. Cooke expressed hope that "no longer will it be possible for physicians, nurses, psychologists, speech and physical therapists to graduate from their respective training programs totally ignorant of the clinical problems of the mentally and physically handicapped."[35] UAF directors wanted their facilities to eventually become prominent enough at universities and medical schools that clinical rotations through them would be included as a standard part of most clinical professional training.

Since many of the initial UAFs and MRRCs were literally built from the ground up with federal construction funds, it was not until the late 1960s that these facilities began to have a major presence on the national level. Over this period and into the 1970s and '80s, pediatricians continued to focus on developing and defining their particular roles within multidisciplinary teams focused on mental retardation and other developmental disabilities. Many pediatricians sought to establish themselves as the preeminent leaders in this area—an ambition that would necessarily involve jurisdictional conflicts with psychiatrists and ongoing engagement with educators, who were also pushing to have a leading role in community-based disability services.

Leadership in Developmental Disabilities

As pediatricians became more interested in children with developmental disabilities during the 1960s, they argued that their professional training, skills, and relationships with families made them uniquely well-suited for being the leading professionals in the area.[36] They were also motivated by the power and prestige that came with this designation. Leadership was not simply theirs for the taking. There were jurisdictional battles to be fought, since most US states recognized psychiatrists as overseeing mental retardation services. Additionally, to become leaders in developmental disabilities, pediatricians would need to expand the expertise and services that they offered families well beyond their existing role in providing the initial diagnosis to also include long-term empathetic support, family guidance, and care-coordination.

Beginning in the early 1960s, NARC and AAP developed a collaborative relationship to help pediatricians expand their leadership in mental retardation services, including residential institutions. As NARC put it, "Some states feel that institutions for the retarded must be staffed primarily, if not exclusively, with psychiatrists. Yet a large percentage of those admitted clearly require the most intensive and comprehensive pediatric program but would not be considered appropriate subjects for psychiatric treatment, were they in the community."[37] Pediatricians, of course, had also contributed to the institutionalization of young children with mental retardation, which many NARC parents strongly rejected. Nonetheless, NARC advocates tended to trust pediatricians much more than psychiatrists, in part due to their common interests in developing parallel services for children with developmental disabilities in local communities.[38] Clinical psychologists often worked in institutional settings as well—assessing IQ, conducting research, and developing training programs. However, as fellow physicians, psychiatrists were pediatricians' primary competitors for leadership roles and recognition by US states and the federal government as the primary authorities overseeing clinical institutions and services.

Cooke was actively involved in challenging psychiatry's control over mental retardation services. He campaigned for oversight of Maryland's mental retardation program, which included two residential institutions, to be shifted from the Department of Mental Hygiene to the Health Department. In a 1963 *Baltimore Sun* article, Cooke argued that mental retardation was "basically a medical problem rather than a psychiatric problem, and its detection, prevention, and treatment is the concern of those in the child health field rather than of psychiatrists." All of Maryland's resources for mental retardation, Cooke complained, went to the Department of Mental Hygiene, which was unnecessarily keeping children in residential institutions overseen by psychiatrists, who had "almost zero" interest in patients with intellectual limitations.[39] Leon Eisenberg, Chief of Child Psychiatry at Johns Hopkins, responded to Cooke's assertions by lamenting the rise of jurisdictional fights in Maryland and other states over mental retardation programs, "now that [federal] funds are becoming available."[40] He preferred a collaborative oversight structure involving the Department of Mental Hygiene and the Health Department.

Disciplinary battles over state jurisdiction continued into the next decade, with psychiatrists in multiple populous US states retaining control of residential institutions for mental retardation. University of Southern California pediatrician Richard Koch acknowledged that the situation was largely a product of the recent past, in which "pediatricians seldom wished to become involved in the care of the mentally retarded in any measure beyond the usual procedures provided for any normal child."[41] Indeed, as Giannini had learned from parents in the 1950s, pediatricians often even denied basic health care to children with mental retardation. A professional jurisdiction that might have come quite naturally to pediatricians had not initially been pursued and was now proving difficult, in many places, to reclaim from psychiatrists.

By the late 1950s, a number of pediatricians were actively defining a leadership role for themselves in developmental disabilities. In 1957, the AAP Committee on the Handicapped Child noted the need to "help prepare and orient pediatricians for the role of 'coordinator' in the field of pediatric rehabilitation," especially in the care of children with neurological disabilities.[42] Two years later, pediatrician Hulda Thelander, who directed the Child Development Center at San Francisco Children's Hospital and specialized in cerebral palsy, mental retardation, and other developmental disabilities, argued, "In the case of a handicapped child the problem is primarily medical. The physician should therefore be at the helm and the agencies and other disciplines should be in an ancillary role." Similarly, in 1960, pediatrician Robert Warner of the Children's Rehabilitation Center in Buffalo, which specialized in mental retardation and cerebral palsy, noted, "The pediatrician is pre-eminent in this setting. . . . All those who have examined the patient meet in professional conference, which is conducted by the pediatrician. The pediatrician also conducts the parent conference."[43] A few years later, a proposal for a multidisciplinary mental retardation center at the University of Washington stated that, "The Medical Director should be a qualified pediatrician," who would "have final authority over all medical care and practice."[44] Indeed, there was a clear sense at many clinics for children with developmental disabilities that a pediatrician should be the face and figurehead of the operation.

Increasing efforts during the late 1960s to move mental retardation services away from residential institutions and instead to community-based locations—including UAFs—offered new leadership opportunities for pediatricians. Among 37 UAF directors in 1973, more than 20 were pediatricians, while ten held PhDs, primarily in psychology, and just one was an EdD.[45] Four of the first five presidents of the Association of University Affiliated Facilities were also pediatricians.[46] While psychiatrists were providers and clinical team members in many UAFs, few had leadership roles. One exception was George Tarjan, who directed the Pacific State Hospital residential institution, which was affiliated with the University of California, Los Angeles. Tarjan was a long-standing and highly regarded leader in the mental retardation area. Some pediatricians, parents, and advocates viewed Tarjan as a rare reformer among psychiatrists.[47]

Beyond jurisdictional battles, pediatricians knew that, to be leaders in developmental disabilities, they also needed to establish good relationships with families and provide ongoing and multifaceted clinical services. Pediatricians were often the first clinicians to examine and diagnose children with mental retardation and other developmental disabilities. However, as AAP's manual *The Pediatrician and the Child with Mental Retardation* (1971) acknowledged, "Historically . . . once the diagnosis and evaluation have been completed, [the pediatrician] has often assumed that his participation in providing ongoing services is at an end."[48] To lead and to enhance their professional prestige in the area of developmental disabilities, pediatricians needed to expand their interests, skills, and services well beyond this perfunctory role. Part of the challenge was in learning how to manage the initial diagnostic encounter in ways that would not discourage and dismay parents such that they sought out other clinicians' opinions and help.

During the 1960s and '70s, many pediatricians who specialized in mental retardation expressed concern about the frequency with which parents re-jected their initial interpretations and advice, and instead went "shopping" around for other diagnoses and services. Pediatricians viewed it as a major waste of professional time and resources when parents went from one pro-vider to the next, seeking a different result. They also worried that some caregivers would willfully exploit desperate parents by promising to help their child with therapies that most pediatricians refused to offer. Certainly, there was a fair share of quackery out there—including unproven, expen-sive, and time-consuming interventions. Mindful of this, pediatricians were sensitive about protecting their domain of expertise as gatekeepers for ef-fective interventions. Some argued that the best way to limit shopping, and its associated ills, was to provide more sympathetic, adequate, and exhaus-tive information to parents at the time of diagnosis.[49]

The American Medical Association's (AMA) 1965 handbook for physi-cians on mental retardation emphasized the significance of physicians pro-viding parents not just with a diagnosis, but also support—with a "flexible attitude" and recognition that the child "may have unrealized potentialities for development." Allowing adequate time for evaluation and planning, the AMA handbook suggested, could help to "minimize parental shopping for other opinions." The handbook editors, led by prominent pediatrician and future Surgeon General Julius Richmond, also encouraged physicians to di-rect parents to support organizations like NARC, which only promoted sci-entifically proven methods and could help to curb diagnosis shopping.[50]

In 1968, Paul Pearson, a pediatrician and director of the University of Nebraska's UAF in Omaha, recommended a multidisciplinary approach to diagnosis and parent counseling. He suggested that "thorough evaluations by a skilled team of specialists also tends to forestall the parents' customary rejection of the diagnosis and the 'shopping' which often follows. However, this is true only if the diagnostic process is followed by adequate education, counseling, and skillful management."[51] Numerous published reports de-scribed the bluntness, indifference, and hopelessness with which many phy-sicians conveyed their diagnosis of mental retardation to parents.[52] Pearson acknowledged that parents were often initially resistant to a mental retar-dation diagnosis. It was part of the physician's job to win their trust by way of a thorough biomedical assessment, as well as empathetic counseling and ongoing support.

Importantly, having been trained within a pediatrics discipline that actively avoided caring for children with developmental disabilities, few pediatricians practicing in the 1960s and '70s were well versed in how to provide a sensitive and supportive disability diagnosis. Many conveyed, either directly or attitudinally, the pessimism of their formative era. Some young pediatricians, when facing their first encounter with developmental disabilities in a newborn or toddler, were shocked by how poorly prepared they were to communicate the diagnosis and properly respond to parents' emotions and concerns. As a second-year resident in pediatrics during the early 1970s, John C. Carey needed to inform parents that their newborn child had Down syndrome. At that moment, he realized that he had no experience, insight, or training for this challenging situation. Carey had been given no basic script, no sense of best practices, and was unprepared for responding to questions about withholding treatments or institutionalization. After a difficult interaction providing the initial diagnosis, Carey was conscious not to avoid the parents. He found that over time they warmed to him and were happy to speak with him in the well-baby clinic after they had fully accepted and integrated this new child into their home.[53]

Many pediatricians in Carey's position were inclined to just give a quick, often very pessimistic diagnosis and then walk away—leaving it to someone else, if the parents were lucky, to provide needed social and emotional support. With the changing politics of the late 1960s, some pediatricians began to take on more activist roles. In 1966, pediatrician Robert Kugel took over as chair of the AAP Committee on the Handicapped Child. At the time, Kugel was establishing himself as a leading reformer in the area of developmental disabilities—particularly with the publication of *Changing Patterns in Residential Services for the Mentally Retarded* (1969), which he coedited with clinical psychologist Wolf Wolfensberger (chapter 1). Under Kugel, the committee changed its name to the Committee on Children with Handicaps (CCWH)—adopting "person-first" language to demonstrate its focus on the child and not the disability. Kugel and his CCWH colleagues further stated that "our responsibility is far greater than just to pediatricians since we have a concern for children . . . whatever their health problems. In developing statements there need not be an attempt to avoid controversy."[54] There was an expressed willingness for CCWH to engage not only in medical considerations, but in sociopolitical topics as well. Foremost among these was the continued institutionalization of disabled children, which pediatricians increasingly opposed—especially before school age.

During Kugel's tenure as chair, CCWH wrote and published AAP's *Pediatrician and the Child with Mental Retardation*, which conveyed the discipline's evolving role and perspectives. Gunnar Dybwad, a prominent disability advocate and former executive director of NARC, was specially acknowledged by the authors for his role in shaping the final product; they noted, "With changing attitudes in recent years, the pediatrician has been called on to provide ongoing counseling to the parents regarding a variety of psycho-socioeducational factors." The proper role for a present-day physician, the authors held, was as the "coordinator of a multidisciplinary team."[55] In addition to medical and other clinical professional aspects of mental retardation, the manual included a few short sections on community services, legal considerations, and the pediatrician's social roles and responsibilities beyond the clinic. On the whole, its focus was primarily clinical, but the authors did seriously address the psychosocial impacts of mental retardation on children and families and the importance of parent advocacy.

The AAP manual also aimed to help pediatricians convince themselves, and the families they consulted, that institutionalization was not the best option for many children with developmental disabilities. In doing so, the authors included a rather hopeful photograph of a young girl with Down syndrome. She wore a nice dress with a bow on her shoulder and her hair carefully styled. The caption noted that she lived at home and was "friendly, well mannered, and well behaved" but then quickly fell into clinical speak, stating, "Her I.Q. is 50. Note the not unattractive appearance and good grooming." Rather than playing or smiling, the young girl was depicted in a stereotypical manner—staring at the camera with her mouth open. The image was not empowering—it did not highlight her interests or strengths, beyond being mild mannered and socially presentable, as fit with the normative expectations for a white, middle-class girl. She was medicalized and objectified, but still there was some effort to offer an optimistic outlook. Here was a young child with Down syndrome who was not institutionalized. She went to a community "nursery school for normal children" and was accepted into "a public school class for trainable, retarded children."[56] This characterization showed significant progress in more positive and inclusive disability narratives, at the same time that it served the interests of the authors. They framed Down syndrome as a medical problem, while encouraging care in a community setting, where pediatricians could lead the ongoing clinical assessment and support.

As pediatricians became more engaged in providing long-term care for children with developmental disabilities, they grew to appreciate that these families had an array of social and medical support needs, which fell into the domains of various other clinicians and professionals. Some questioned whether these services were being adequately provided and coordinated, and identified a role for pediatricians in the ongoing oversight of this care. As Constance Battle put it, pediatricians should play the role of "ombudsman" in the health care of handicapped children. Early in her pediatrics career, Battle's daughter Ursula was born with cerebral palsy. This event motivated Battle to shift her professional ambitions from running a private practice out of her home to taking on administrative leadership positions within health care institutions.[57]

In 1972, Battle wrote about the potential shortcomings of team-based care and the importance of having one person always designated as the co-ordinator. She suggested that "it is the logical role of the pediatrician to assume responsibility and leadership of the team." Battle offered further specificity on the pediatrician's role, stating, "The responsibility of the pediatric ombudsman would be to review all aspects of the child's functioning, not only with the specialists caring for him, but also with his family, school, and community."[58] The pediatrician's leadership role would thus extend beyond their professional office, specialty clinic, or hospital and intersect with community-based educational and social services. In practice, a pediatrician's care would also sometimes extend beyond the childhood years, since no adult medical discipline claimed a specialty jurisdiction in developmental disabilities in the 1970s—or to the present day.

The next year, a team of pediatricians at the University of Rochester who were studying multidisciplinary care teams for children with spina bifida specifically looked for evidence that pediatricians were engaging in Battle's "ombudsman" role. Parents surveyed for their study did not feel that any one of their physicians was taking primary responsibility for the comprehensive care of their child with spina bifida. Rather, they believed that their primary physicians were insufficiently knowledgeable about spina bifida or the available community resources for their children. Families also highlighted that specialists and specialty clinics generally did not provide standard well-child care—some parents had anticipated that they would. In all, only 18 percent of the parents suggested that their child was receiving comprehensive oversight from a single provider. The authors concluded that neither general pediatricians nor specialists were playing Battle's ombudsman role for the great majority of the 44 families surveyed. They suggested that specialty clinics or community agencies should designate a "coordinating physician" for families, since primary care pediatricians were not showing active leadership in taking on this role.[59]

Indeed, into the 1970s, pediatricians' talk of leadership and care-coordination for children with developmental disabilities and their families was often more aspirational than consistently implemented. During this period, pediatrician Siegfried Pueschel and social worker Ann Murphy at Boston Children's Hospital were actively engaged in studying and providing a new model for pediatric care in the developmental disabilities area. Based on analysis of hundreds of parent interviews and questionnaires, Pueschel and Murphy concluded in a 1975 article,

> Telling new parents that their baby has Down's syndrome takes a high degree of skill and sensitivity. What is said—and when, how, and by whom—will greatly influence the child's chances of being raised in a nurturing environment.... The physician should emphasize that the infant with Down's syndrome is first and foremost a human being with characteristics apart from the stereotype and with inherent rights.[60]

Physicians, they argued, needed to offer parents information, hope, empowerment, and a clear sense of what resources their family deserved. Pueschel and Murphy's research highlighted the importance of the initial diagnostic encounter for families—noting that it should be viewed as the beginning of parents' adjustment to their child's disabilities and of the pediatrician's caring role, rather than as an isolated event.

In addressing Down syndrome, Pueschel also spoke from his own personal experience. His son Christian, who was born in 1965, had Down syndrome. As part of Pueschel's efforts to better advocate clinically and socially for Christian and other disabled individuals, he would eventually earn a master's in public health, a PhD in psychology, and a law degree. Over his career, he coauthored numerous books on Down syndrome, written for both clinician and parent audiences, which incorporated a wide variety of perspectives and voices, on medical, social, and legal aspects.[61]

Along with Cooke, Battle, and a number of other postwar pediatricians who had family members with developmental disabilities, Pueschel played an influential role in describing and demonstrating a leadership role for pediatrics in this area. Along the way, he also achieved a very successful, prestigious, and multifaceted career in clinical care and research—first as the director of a Down syndrome clinic at Boston Children's Hospital and later as the director of the UAF at Brown University. Similar opportunities for professional advancement and recognition in pediatrics, while specializing in developmental disabilities, had been much less widely available before the 1960s.

For many postwar pediatricians, passion for working with children and families with developmental disabilities—whatever its origins—was mixed up with considerations of role, status, and career advancement. In their efforts to claim jurisdiction, pediatricians presented developmental disabilities as a medical—and not a mental health—problem, which was best addressed in community settings like UAFs and private practices, where they had greater control and influence. As part of this, pediatricians presented highly stigmatized conditions like Down syndrome as manageable in the home and not necessarily disruptive of the ideals of middle-class family life. They also increasingly recognized the degree to which the initial diagnosis was an important starting point for developing a more positive, optimistic, and informed parent-child relationship, as well as a key moment in building a physician-family bond. If pediatricians were to be leaders in developmental disabilities, these connections needed to be nurtured. Otherwise, parents would look elsewhere. Indeed, even as pediatricians improved their diagnostic and care-coordination skills, they faced multiple competitors for leadership in developmental disabilities.

Challenges to Pediatrics Leadership

In the 1960s, Robert Cooke's close personal and professional relationships with the Kennedy family brought the perspectives and interests of pediatricians to the center of American political power. During the 1970s and '80s, this was no longer the case. In fact, by this time, pediatricians were actively falling behind in influencing the US government's evolving policies related to children with developmental disabilities. Initially, pediatricians had little idea that this was the even case. However, it became acutely apparent with the passage of the Education for All Handicapped Children Act (PL 94-142) in 1975. This legislation drastically enhanced the rights and the guaranteed public educational services available for disabled children. The

Act mandated that all children from age three to 21 receive a free and developmentally appropriate education in the most inclusive possible setting within their community schools.[62]

When pediatricians reviewed the legislation, they noted to their dismay that no explicit role for them had been included. In an assessment of the law published after its implementation had already begun, pediatrician Judith Palfrey and colleagues stated:

> In many ways P.L. 94-142 marks a shift in emphasis away from the so-called "medical model" to the less traditional "educational model." It is somewhat telling that the responsibilities of education agencies are clearly defined under P.L. 94-142, but the responsibilities of medical professionals are not well delineated at all. This lack of definition . . . reflects a basic ambivalence about the role of the health professionals in the special-education process.[63]

While some states in their implementation protocols did continue to require pediatricians' involvement in individualized educational planning, the expectation in most places was that physicians would be consulted exclusively on an "as-needed" basis.[64]

The language of PL 94-142 was a significant blow to pediatricians' efforts to establish a leadership role in developmental disabilities. Congress had come down definitively on the side of educators in the debate over whether disability should primarily be addressed through medical or educational interventions. Pediatricians' lack of familiarity with the Act before it was passed—and the fact that the original bill referred to only one medical field, child neurology—was interpreted as evidence that the bill's authors had actively avoided the input of physicians. As CCWH noted, while many child neurologists *could* technically fulfill their assigned role in examining children for learning disabilities, it was obvious that child neurology lacked the workforce numbers for this. Also, most of its practitioners had little interest in the area (chapter 5).[65]

In 1976, as the drafting of regulations for PL 94-142 was underway, Richard Masland—himself a neurologist and a previous research director for NARC—asked CCWH to help influence the regulatory process. He was "distressed to learn of the absence of medical input."[66] CCWH considered submitting a statement on the proper make up for a disability diagnosis and evaluation team—at the most basic level a physician (preferably a pediatrician), psychologist, educator, and audiology/speech specialist. Ultimately, the committee failed to reach consensus on the issue. As a result, AAP did not send any official comments on the regulations.[67]

By and large, the opportunity to influence federal policy in PL 94-142 had already evaporated before pediatricians even noticed what was happening. Over the previous decade, CCWH had occasionally discussed the need for improved engagement with educators, and their concern that "educators usually don't recognize pediatricians in the field of education."[68] These calls for reaching out and improving relations went unheeded. Following the passage of PL 94-142—without any input from pediatricians—CCWH commented that "the 'Educators' are well organized and have actively sought and obtained control over the various education programs impacting upon the handicapped. Steps must be taken toward more cooperative relations between the health and education sectors."[69] In 1977, as the PL 94-142 regulations were being finalized, CCWH member Robert Stempfel testified before Congress. CCWH noted that his was the first of sixteen hearings to include testimony from a physician.[70] While pediatricians believed that a leadership role in developmental disabilities was appropriate for their field, the necessary political oversight, action, and collaboration for this to be achieved clearly had not taken place.

The final rules for PL 94-142 were published in the Federal Register in August 1977. Frustrated conversations among pediatricians about their exclusion lasted for years thereafter.[71] Even with some late-stage lobbying, no mandate to include a physician on disability evaluation teams was included in the Act. CCWH attributed this outcome to the law's privileging of educational over medical approaches, as well as the costs associated with including physicians.[72] Compensation for evaluations related to PL 94-142 was a major concern for pediatricians. Because medical assessments were listed in the Act as a "related service," there was no funding included to help pay for them. Also, when medical opinions were requested by school systems, there was some concern that third-party payers would refuse to compensate for them and assert that money should come from the federal government. Ultimately, even as the care and oversight of children with developmental disabilities was rapidly moving from residential institutions into local communities during the 1970s, pediatricians found that other professionals—this time educators rather than psychiatrists—had managed to preemptively claim government-mandated priority, jurisdiction, influence, and compensation in this expert domain.

Pediatric disability specialists perceived additional professional threats after the 1980 election of Ronald Reagan. Before Reagan was even inaugurated, CCWH members expressed serious concerns about changes to federal allocations, which would affect care and research related to disabled children.[73] Reagan's election also reflected and fomented the rise of pro-life politics, with potential impacts on the recent uptake of prenatal testing and selective abortion to prevent Down syndrome and other disabilities (chapter 6).[74] Beyond access to abortion, the pro-life movement under Reagan also focused on the care of newborn disabled children. There had long been opposition to the hands-off approach that some physicians adopted in these cases, such as withholding treatment to see if a newborn infant would survive on its own, as well as passively accepting parents' directives to forgo operations to save the life of their disabled child.

Robert Cooke and Eunice Kennedy Shriver played an influential role in bringing cases of withholding treatment from newborn disabled children to public attention. Most notable was their film *Who Should Survive?* (1971), which reenacted a case from Johns Hopkins, where parents refused a gastrointestinal surgery and allowed their newborn with Down syndrome to die of starvation in the hospital. The reenactment was followed by a discussion involving Cooke, sociologist Renée Fox, and multiple field-founding bioethicists.[75] A number of the physicians that I interviewed had viewed this film during their training or had shown it to students (as I do today).

During the 1970s, Cooke engaged with and critiqued the fledgling field of bioethics' pessimistic and dismissive views of childhood disability. In a 1972 *Journal of Pediatrics* editorial, Cooke challenged the common refrain that choosing lifesaving interventions for newborns with "severe" disabilities only led to unnecessary "suffering." He argued that these were relative interpretations, put forward by nondisabled physicians and ethicists who had experienced life without a "severe" condition. Inevitably, what these adults interpreted as unacceptable "suffering" was colored by their own experiences.[76]

In the early 1980s, the Reagan Administration chose to take political action against withholding treatment from newborns by announcing a new interpretation of Section 504 of the 1973 Rehabilitation Act (chapter 1), which guaranteed access to federally funded institutions for disabled people. This effort to change federal regulations came to be known as the "Baby Doe Rules." The Administration threatened hospitals with loss of Federal funding in cases where life-sustaining treatments were not provided for newborn disabled children. Signs were posted in hospitals, and hotlines were set up to facilitate the reporting of cases by hospital staff.

Pediatricians—while sensitive to the problematic nature of withholding treatment simply to "prevent" disability—were strongly opposed to such federal involvement in difficult decisions made in the context of "severely" affected newborns. AAP acknowledged that the new rule was "clearly intended to remind health care professionals and hospitals that they are obligated to avoid discrimination against the handicapped in the delivery of health care services," but the AAP opposed blunt federal incursion as the right approach for solving what was a long-standing and complex problem. Medical intervention, AAP argued, was not always in the best interests of patients, and withholding treatment was frequently justified for both legal and ethical reasons.[77]

The infiltration of national politics into the doctor-patient relationship was a matter of serious concern for pediatricians, especially when it interfered with deeply personal and difficult decisions. Still, pediatricians recognized that times were changing, and the laissez-faire status quo of past decades, which had allowed newborn disabled children to die in the back wards of hospitals at their parents' request, was no longer acceptable. Over time, deinstitutionalization, improved early intervention programs, and guaranteed public education helped to demonstrate that many children with developmental disabilities had greater potential than was previously assumed. Also, the widespread uptake of new surgeries greatly increased the life expectancy of individuals with Down syndrome, who were often born with heart defects.[78] Ultimately, Congress codified some of the intentions of the Baby Doe Rules in 1984 revisions to the Child Abuse Act, making violations enforceable by states instead of the US federal government.

New legislation and federal rule-making related to disabled children during the 1970s and '80s reflected broader sociopolitical trends, which pediatricians increasingly acknowledged and respected. Nonetheless, they felt threatened by the shifting landscape of government involvement in health care regulation and funding. Pediatricians were no longer playing a leading role in political conversations about how to better support children with developmental disabilities, as they had when the Kennedy Administration had readily turned to Cooke for advice. Amid these changes, pediatricians were developing new approaches, such as the medical home concept, that established their role in holistic care and helped make the case for better funding.

The Medical Home Concept

In 1974, University of Rochester pediatrician Robert Haggerty called for more sustained interest in what he called the "new morbidity" in pediatrics, which included chronic physical disorders, violence, substance use, teen pregnancy, and child abuse. The transition required pediatricians to become more active in their local communities, engaging with factors that could not be readily observed from their offices.[79] This shift was particularly relevant to caring for children with developmental disabilities, whose access to community-based resources, schooling, and acceptance was quickly evolving at this time. As part of this, the 1967 edition of AAP's *Standards of Child Health Care* stated, "For children with chronic diseases or disabling conditions, the lack of a complete record and a 'medical home' is a major deterrent to adequate health supervision."[80] A child's medical records were often spread across many institutions, including their pediatrician, emergency rooms, specialists, physicians in other cities, and schools. AAP believed that the active consolidation of disabled children's medical records and care coordination within a single primary care "medical home" would lead to significant improvement in outcomes. Importantly, over the coming decades, AAP expanded this medical home concept to illustrate the best practices in community-based primary care for *all* children.

Pediatrician Calvin Sia was a particularly prominent champion of the medical home concept as it developed into a fully formed model of care-coordination. Sia, a primary care pediatrician in Honolulu, was a strong proponent of pediatricians' advocacy role in bringing about and institutionalizing change at the local, state, and national levels—including the improvement of schools and government welfare programs. As part of this, in 1978 he organized a gathering of government and medical officials in Hawaii to "design an integrated system of services that would assure every child a medical home where they could receive primary health care services addressing the needs of the whole child." The plan included Sia's phrase, "Every child deserves a medical home," which became one of AAP's central goals for child health.[81]

As it evolved in the 1980s, AAP defined the medical home approach as "a method of providing primary care from a community level, recognizing the importance of addressing the needs of the total child and family in relationship to health, education, family support, and the social environment."[82] The concept was similar to Constance Battle's call for pediatricians to play the role of "ombudsman" in overseeing the wide-ranging care of disabled children in the community. While such ambitions were not readily achieved in the 1970s, by the 1990s, the medical home concept gave new life and interest to Battle's "total care" model for pediatrics.[83] Importantly, the medical home concept encouraged that these more wide-ranging services be a part of all pediatric primary care, in addition to noting their value for disabled individuals.

AAP's first official statement on the medical home, in 1992, described it as "accessible, continuous, comprehensive, family centered, coordinated, and compassionate."[84] Primary care pediatricians would set up and maintain a child's medical home, which included oversight of child development, outpatient and inpatient care, specialists, schools, and community agencies. While the pediatrician could not always be physically present, they were to act as "the child's advocate and assume control and ultimate responsibility to the care that is provided."[85] Childhood disability specialists responded very favorably to the comprehensive nature of the medical home approach and its characterization of pediatricians as team leaders. The recently renamed AAP Committee on Children with Disabilities (CCWD) also embraced the medical home concept's emphasis on family-centered care, noting that families should "participate in the management of their child's care in a cooperative effort rather than as subordinates."[86]

CCWD's investment in promoting family-led care was further demonstrated by its choice, in 1995, to newly include a member who represented a parent advocacy group. For many years, CCWD had a liaison relationship with The Arc (formerly NARC), but this representative was always a physician. The new parent advocate, from the organization Family Voices, was invited to provide "the 'family' perspective regarding disability issues."[87] Family Voices was a particularly good fit for this collaboration because the group focused on health care issues broadly and represented children with various forms of disability. Its formal relations with the CCWD were long lasting and productive, especially on medical home issues related to disability.

Within AAP, the Medical Home Project working group was highly collaborative, bringing together various contingencies within the Association to work toward common goals.[88] Cooperation proved important during the Clinton Administration's push for comprehensive health care reform, especially when policies affected disabled children and those with other special needs—who at times required uniquely intensive or time-consuming services.[89] Notably, during the 1990s, AAP's advocacy on behalf of disabled children otherwise suffered from a lack of coordination, due to significant tensions among various disability interest groups (chapter 5). In this context, the Medical Home Project offered valuable opportunities for engagement on disability issues, keeping the focus on advocacy for children rather than professional concerns.

Despite the concept's broad adoption within AAP, many primary care pediatricians were hesitant to adopt a medical home model for their own private practice, due to its anticipated costs and the presumed difficulty in receiving sufficient compensation from insurers.[90] Extended office visits and care-coordination were not well represented in insurance coding schemes, nor always approved by third-party payers, who were much more familiar with, and supportive of, short consultations and discrete medical procedures. In 2012, the AAP Committee on Child Health Financing stated, "Overall, the fee-for-service system is proving to be an inadequate mechanism for funding to support the core elements of the family-centered medical home."[91] These financial challenges were particularly acute for pediatricians seeking to provide a comprehensive medical home, which would include community support and care-coordination for disabled children.

During the 2000s, pediatrician W. Carl Cooley took the lead in developing guidelines and advice on how to provide a medical home for disabled children. He had both clinical and personal experience in the area—his daughter Sarah has Down syndrome. Cooley highlighted the importance of scheduling extra time when disabled children made office visits, noted that any physical barriers to movement within the office needed be evaluated and addressed for wheelchair users, and recommended that written care plans should be developed and reviewed with family members. Cooley also provided an overview of coding and reimbursement options for medical home services and support involving children with developmental disabilities, although he acknowledged that public and private insurers frequently denied these codes.[92]

During the 1990s, AAP developed the medical home concept into an effective means of articulating pediatricians' leadership role and responsibilities in managing broad-based care for all children—including those with disabilities. A 2008 study concluded that a medical home was likely to improve child health and family support outcomes for children with special heath care needs. The authors noted that, while the medical home concept did not differ significantly from the ideals of primary care, the rebranding did seem to improve the available resources—through special grants and organizational funding—for care-coordination and planning. This was an important finding, especially given that debt-burdened medical students often regarded primary care "as undervalued with relatively lower incomes, longer work hours, [and] less prestige."[93]

The medical home concept proved very productive for pediatricians as they sought to define and improve the professional status and compensation associated with caring for children with developmental disabilities. It provided a justification for extending the reach of pediatric services and oversight into community agencies and offered a new language and billing codes to argue for improved compensation for the sometimes intensive and multifaceted care that they provided to disabled children and their families. Notably, the medical home concept also represented a model of total care for *all* children, which—in its ideal application—could be particularly valuable for those who had developmental disabilities or other chronic conditions.

Conclusions

During the postwar period, many pediatricians, who—for a variety of reasons—had developed a vocation in providing care and support to children with developmental disabilities and their families, began looking for ways to improve the respectability, status, and opportunities associated with this long-overlooked and dismissed area. Specialists in childhood disability believed that new pathways for career advancement and better compensation would benefit them professionally and also help attract more young physicians to pursue training or research on developmental disabilities. Robert Cooke, in particular, recognized and promoted the idea that encouraging greater passion *through enhanced prestige* was an effective strategy for improving the quality of research and care in developmental disabilities, while addressing workforce needs.

Appeals to pediatricians' unique leadership potential in developmental disabilities were another key part of the campaign to enhance prestige and respect for practitioners who worked in this area. Efforts in this direction involved presenting developmental disabilities as primarily a "medical problem," best addressed by pediatricians through clinical research and interventions, as well as broad-based care coordination. This viewpoint proved to have serious limitations in the 1970s, as pediatricians struggled to gain a leadership foothold. Even as their commitment and investment in children with developmental disabilities grew, and jurisdictional competition from psychiatrists began to fall away, pediatricians clearly remained out of touch—especially with evolving legislative trends and available community resources. Amid this, pediatricians whose own children had developmental disabilities were particularly powerful and influential leaders for the discipline. They uniquely encouraged greater engagement with sociopolitical disability advocacy, while also promoting more comprehensive models of practice for pediatric care.

Larger postwar trends in pediatrics, involving the "new morbidity" and "medical home" concept, offered novel ways for professionals to consider and frame their leadership efforts in developmental disabilities—including broader roles in community services and outreach. The medical home model also helped pediatricians establish new strategies for requesting adequate compensation for services outside of acute interventions and well-child care. The fact that the medical home concept was intended for *all* children, while also being uniquely valuable for the total care of those with disabilities, aided the likelihood for its widespread uptake. Indeed, as disability scholar and self-advocate Irving Zola has argued, when policies that support disabled individuals also benefit people more universally, they have much greater long-term potential.[94]

Postwar pediatricians' perspectives and advocacy related to disability were quite distinct from many of the clinical psychologists that I highlighted in chapter 1. This was largely because pediatricians' patients were almost exclusively young children. Clinical psychologists, especially those who specialized in physical disabilities, most often worked with adults. Some psychologists were also disabled themselves. No similar, practitioner-led self-advocacy movement existed in postwar pediatrics (although some visibly disabled practitioners entered the discipline and engaged in advocacy in the 2000s[95]). The disability advocates who most actively influenced late twentieth-century pediatricians were parents. In clinical psychology, disability self-advocates pushed for new efforts to overcome the social and professional discrimination that impacted disabled adults, who were living independently in their communities and pursuing careers. Whereas, disability advocacy in pediatrics was much more oriented toward the concerns of families and nondisabled professionals—concerns about the availability of community services, inclusion in public schools, and opportunities for pediatrics career advancement. Pediatricians thus had more in common with psychologists who specialized in intellectual disabilities, a topic I examine in chapters 4 and 5.

Meanwhile, chapter 3 turns to the parallel history of postwar genetic counseling—a field of clinical professionals who frequently worked closely alongside pediatricians in caring for children and families with developmental disabilities. Some genetic counselors pushed their field toward a broader role in disability advocacy beyond the clinical setting. However, as with pediatrics and clinical psychology, the professional identity and prestige associated with more narrowly focusing on research, expertise, and practice with individual patients discouraged genetic counselors from making the leap into sociopolitical and community advocacy roles.

3

Genetic Counseling

Identity and Role in a New Clinical Field

In 1972, Joan Marks a psychiatric social worker became the codirector of the first master's training program in genetic counseling, located at Sarah Lawrence College. Marks's initial survey of the program and its clinical training sites revealed a strong focus on communicating genetic and medical information for the purposes of achieving logical decision-making and carefully avoiding any "emotional responses" among patients or genetic counselors. Marks concluded that the counseling component of the program was seriously deficient and believed that trainees should be taught to approach their patients "not as receptacles of genetic information, but as people in a crisis."[1] This would require more training in counseling skills, which were not initially part of the program's curriculum. Counseling could be taught in the clinic, but Marks believed that the "medical model" dominated at the program's clinical training sites. So, she decided to incorporate counseling skills into classroom instruction, beginning with a new course taught by a psychotherapist. Sarah Lawrence's commitment to teaching more advanced counseling skills and psychodynamic perspectives grew from there. Decades later, these elements were still regarded as the program's distinguishing features.[2]

Before the Sarah Lawrence training program was founded, genetic counseling was a specialty area dominated by a small group of (mostly male) physicians and PhD geneticists. During the 1970s and '80s, fifteen master's level training programs were created in the United States and primarily attracted women as students. This transformed the field of genetic counseling into a female-dominated profession, with very few doctoral-trained professionals (whom I refer to as medical geneticists). Initially, MD and PhD medical geneticists were very resistant to the argument that master's trained clinicians possessed enough clinical and scientific knowledge to provide genetic counseling services. Over time, though, they grew to appreciate the many clinical contributions of these new professionals, and their initial opposition dissipated.[3]

Genetic counselors were quite successful in demonstrating their clinical and scientific knowledge. At the same time, physicians who hired them were particularly impressed by their communication skills. As sociologist Regina Kenen put it, "Many medical geneticists realized that genetic counseling involved a psychologically oriented approach and therapeutic techniques that were not part of their medical training."[4] While up-to-date knowledge of clinical genetics was fundamental to the professional acceptance of genetic counselors, their ability to convey complex and emotionally difficult information greatly contributed to their indispensability.

This chapter examines the history of the master's level genetic counseling field since its establishment in the 1970s. My analysis throughout this chapter is informed by the work of historians Alexandra Stern, Nathaniel Comfort, and Devon Stillwell, who have insightfully addressed many aspects of this history in great detail, including the relevance of eugenics, gender, and race in genetic counseling.[5] However, I touch upon these important topics only in passing, but I strongly encourage your engagement with their incisive scholarship in this area as well. My focus is on the development, and competing visions of, professional identity and role in genetic counseling. Most late twentieth-century genetic counselors, along with their national organization, emphasized their professional roles as biomedical educators and empathetic communicators, as well as clinically based advocates for individual patients and families. These investments led genetic counselors to maintain more individually and pathologically oriented views of disability, which fit comfortably with the perspectives and approaches of physicians and most other health professionals. Meanwhile, disability advocates from outside of the clinical professions suggested that genetic counselors often had little more than a textbook knowledge of disabilities and placed too much emphasis on genetic and clinical aspects of these conditions.[6]

A small number of postwar genetic counselors did help to actively promote more positive and accepting narratives of disability in the clinic, as well as in their communities. Some were involved with support groups for genetic conditions—genetic counselors assisted in producing or reviewing new-parent informational materials that offered more diverse and hopeful perspectives on life with disabilities. Colleagues in their profession sometimes criticized these genetic counselors for validating supposedly overly optimistic portraits of conditions, which were widely perceived to be "severe" or lethal. Importantly, these genetic counselors helped to raise attention and give greater legitimacy to the personal experiences of disabled individuals and their families.

In this chapter, I argue that forces both internal and external to genetic counseling encouraged most practitioners to limit their professional identity and role to disseminating biomedical knowledge and engaging in clinically based advocacy for individual patients. Few late twentieth-century genetic counselors believed that in-depth awareness of the experiences of disabled individuals outside of the clinic—or an identity for the field that centered community-based disability advocacy—represented important components of their practice and expertise.

Genetic counselors often presented their relatively new field as a work in progress. As part of this, some training program directors sought to improve their students' empathy, self-awareness, communication, and counseling skills, especially in comparison to the previous generation of medical geneticists.[7] Nonetheless, blind spots remained in the field's consideration of disability advocacy perspectives. Few genetic counselors accepted or promoted disability advocates' vocal concerns that prenatal diagnosis—in which the field was deeply invested—reified negative, stigmatizing, and discriminatory views of disabled people. Champions of more positive and inclusive views of disability were rare in late twentieth-century genetic counseling—even in comparison to clinical psychology and pediatrics. I know of no disability self-advocates in the profession during most of this period, and I know of only a few parent advocates.[8] As I describe, genetic counseling evolved in various ways during its early decades, but there were only isolated efforts within the field to adopt and promote more positive, accepting, and sociopolitical perspectives on the experiences and possibilities of disabled people.

Building a Professional Identity

Joan Marks took over as director of the first genetic counseling master's degree program a few years after it was founded. Melissa Richter, the dean of graduate studies at Sarah Lawrence College, located just outside of

New York City, had developed the program in 1969. Richter had a background in biology and psychology and a strong interest in women's continuing education. She had envisioned genetic counseling as primarily attracting married women who were returning to school. This demographic made up the majority of the program's early cohorts. In 1972, while Richter was on sabbatical leave, Joan Marks was brought on as codirector. She went on to lead the program for 26 years, after Richter died of breast cancer.[9]

The training program that Marks inherited had a strong biomedical orientation. Its original curriculum consisted of only genetics, medicine, and statistics courses—aside from one seminar taught by a psychiatrist. Since Sarah Lawrence did not have a medical school of its own, the program was dependent on relationships with medical geneticists located in the New York area to train its students clinically. Richter had successfully attracted a number of highly regarded MD and PhD practitioners to participate, but Marks believed that an important dimension of genetic counseling—responding to the patient's immediate psychosocial needs and emotions—was missing. She began by recruiting a psychotherapist to teach a required course on psychodynamic concepts in genetic counseling, which would train counselors to help their patients "'open up' to risk." A few years later, a course on client-centered counseling was also added, to teach students nondirective and client-centered interviewing skills, based on the practices of Carl Rogers.[10]

During the early 1970s, as five more master's training programs in genetic counseling opened across the United States, PhD and MD medical geneticists—who had been calling themselves genetic counselors for decades—took notice. Charles Epstein, a leading and influential pediatric medical geneticist at the University of California, San Francisco, initially objected to master's trained practitioners referring to themselves as genetic counselors, believing that this term should be reserved for physicians. Epstein was not opposed to new allied health professionals developing expertise in genetics and contributing to clinical teams led by pediatricians, but he argued the term *genetic counselor* implied a level of service that could only be provided by properly trained physicians. As he put it, "Associates, aides, collaborators, yes; counselors, no!"[11] At first, Richter and Marks were willing to accept this distinction. In a 1976 *American Journal of Public Health* article, they introduced the new field, referring to their graduates as "genetic associates."[12] The term fit comfortably into the expanding model of allied health professionals and physician extenders, especially since the vast majority of genetic associates were women.[13]

Many early genetic counselors were not satisfied by the diminutive label of *associate*. When master's trained practitioners began organizing to form a national society in the late 1970s, they had to decide what professional title to formally adopt. Given the relative youth of the field, there was some reticence among the participants about choosing a term that many prominent medical geneticists, who were in some cases their supervisors, were openly opposed to sharing. Nonetheless, "genetic counselor" seemed to best capture their training and expertise and did not come with the connotation of a subservient role. As Audrey Heimler, the first president of the National Society of Genetic Counselors (NSGC), later put it, "With some trepidation, given the above history, the By-Laws Committee decided in favor of what they view as the strongest position: graduates of master's degree training programs were equipped to provide genetic counseling, and should be called 'genetic counselors.'"[14] In a second bold move, the By-Laws Committee, composed of nine women who all had genetic counseling master's degrees from Sarah Lawrence, decided that full membership in the organization would be reserved for master's and PhD professionals with training or experience in genetic counseling. Physician medical geneticists could only be nonvoting associate members of NSGC.[15]

Epstein and other physician medical geneticists responded to the NSGC bylaws with significant displeasure. In 1979, Epstein wrote, "I have already been told that because I do not possess the appropriate training and credentials in counseling, I am not a genetic counselor at all. A medical geneticist— yes; a counselor—no!"[16] It was a striking turnaround for physicians who had for decades claimed the term and identity of genetic counselors. While they were not allowed full membership in NSGC, physician medical geneticists retained significant influence over the field because genetic counselors did not have independent mechanisms for professional certification or state-sanctioned licensure. Many genetic counselors continued to work under the direction of MD and PhD medical geneticists, including one physician who expressed concern that NSGC would end up acting more like a labor union than a professional organization.[17]

In short order, many physicians were won over by what genetic counselors could offer. Epstein soon acknowledged, "All who deal with patients in a genetic counseling situation must be concerned with communication, feelings, and the solving of personal problems—*all* must be genetic counselors."[18] He and other medical geneticists were satisfied to retain physician control over making complex genetic diagnoses, while sharing the "psychological aspects of counseling" with other team members. Indeed, beyond being genetics experts, genetic counselors were expected to take on a significant share of the "emotional labor" of patient interactions—a role often left to women.[19] In his ethnographic study of genetic counseling during the late 1970s, sociologist Charles Bosk observed this trend and described how medical geneticists—even though most were male physicians—were regarded as low-status members of their clinical team, and were left with the "mop up" work of managing patients' emotions and frustrations. It is hardly surprising that many medical geneticists happily off-loaded some of these responsibilities onto the rapidly expanding contingent of (mostly female) master's trained genetic counselors.[20]

During the field's first decade, many physicians treated their genetic counselors more like administrative assistants than clinical professionals. In fact, the small proportion of men who did receive master's degrees in the field during its first decade sometimes had trouble finding a job—in part because employers had intended to hire a woman and pay a lower salary.[21] Robin Bennett, who trained at Sarah Lawrence and took a position in medical genetics at the University of Washington, recounted that she was initially treated as a "glorified secretary," who scheduled appointments, assisted physicians during their medical history-taking and clinical exams, and called patients with results. Not surprisingly, a number of early genetic counselors eventually left their positions to pursue further training in medical school or a PhD program. Bennett, on the other hand, established a significant role for herself in patient care, including engagement with patients at the beginning or end of the clinical consultation and taking a family history before the physician entered the room.[22] Bonnie LeRoy, who trained at Sarah Lawrence, was hired by the University of Minnesota on a grant to establish genetic services throughout the state. During her first years on the job, LeRoy convinced multiple physicians at the university that they would benefit from genetic counseling services. Within a decade, she had founded a training program.[23]

When prenatal diagnosis began to expand in the late 1970s, genetic counselors were also hired by obstetricians—who often had little genetics knowledge themselves—to provide risk statistics and counseling before and after amniocentesis. Prenatal testing was a major boon for the field of genetic counseling in the 1980s, creating many new positions and more autonomy, since counselors were often left alone with pregnant couples (chapter 6). Nonetheless, some genetic counselors and medical geneticists, who were active before prenatal diagnosis dominated the field, came to lament the ways in which this trend put a much greater focus on the specific risks of testing and its genetic results rather than on counseling. The ability to do a test and actively respond to its findings—as in the case of amniocentesis and selective abortion to prevent Down syndrome—distracted from deeper discussions with patients about their feelings and perceptions about genetic risk and disability.[24] Genetic counselors who had trained in the 1970s retained an awareness of the era before many genetic tests were available, when counseling was much more about sitting with patients as they contemplated the meaning of genetic uncertainty for themselves and their families. By the 1980s, many patients came in specifically for amniocentesis.

Some genetic counselors during the 1970s and '80s viewed themselves as "pioneering" people, who were passionate about entering an area with unclear career prospects and building a new profession from the ground up.[25] Bennett suggested to me—and there exists significant evidence to back her up—that Marks chose strong women for the Sarah Lawrence program, women who would greatly expand the roles and reach of the field.[26] Indeed, training program directors had significant influence in shaping the direction of genetic counseling in the late twentieth century—through the educational experiences they offered and as gatekeepers of who was accepted into their small, highly competitive graduate programs. Genetic counseling attracted many groundbreaking leaders, but its professional demographics were homogeneous—white, middle-class women, often with undergraduate degrees in biology or psychology. Early program directors did a lot to define the expertise and ambitions of genetic counselors as biomedical experts with strong communication skills. As I describe in the sections ahead, when the profession faced external critiques, there was strong internal resistance to breaking this mold.

Genetic Counselors and Disability Advocacy

In 1979, genetic counselor Carolyn Bay wrote about her nearly two years of involvement with a disability support group for parents of multiply-handicapped children called REACH OUT (Reassurance, Encouragement, Adjustment, Concern, Hope). She noted,

> I personally use the group and the meetings as an opportunity to follow up the families from our clinic and to provide long term genetic counseling. By attending meetings, it is much easier for me to learn the needs of each couple and give them any advice I have to offer. With the trust that time builds, the parents find it much easier to ask questions.[27]

Bay's interactions with REACH OUT were a notable—and quite atypical— example of early genetic counselors actively following families out of the clinic and into the community, to learn more about their challenges, needs, and questions.

Bay's report, in the newly founded *Perspectives in Genetic Counseling* professional newsletter, was one of just a few accounts of real-world engagement with parent support and disability advocacy groups by genetic counselors during the publication's first decade. The most significant contributor to disability coverage in the newsletter during the 1980s was Beth Fine, a genetic counselor at Children's Memorial Hospital in Omaha, who served as the Resources editor of the newsletter. In 1982, Fine noted that, "Genetic counselors are often in a position to inform parents that their child is or will be physically or mentally handicapped. After this initial crisis, genetic counselors assist parents in grieving for the normal child they expected, while helping them to cope with the special needs of their infant."[28] She also highlighted her belief in the central role of genetic counselors in offering postdiagnostic disability services, stating, "The genetic counselor is often the only professional that parents of a disabled child see. Increasingly their problems encompass more than concerns regarding diagnosis, prognosis, and recurrence risk."[29] In Fine's view, the practice of genetic counselors stretched beyond clinical meetings with parents to include long-term advocacy and the provision of support in the wider community.

Fine followed a nontraditional path into genetic counseling. She mostly learned by observing medical geneticists in research and clinical settings. Because there was no training program available in the Omaha area, she earned a master's degree in counseling instead. Medical geneticist Mark Lubinsky, a supervisor of hers, believed that Fine was "born to a be a genetic counselor."[30] She went on to found and direct a new training program at Northwestern University in 1990, which included a specific course on disability. In

Chicago, Fine also got to know Carol J. Gill, a psychologist, disability scholar, and self-advocate (chapter 1). They collaborated on research examining disability perspectives on genetic testing. Genetic counselor Robert Resta recalled that Fine "reached out to the disability community more so than other people did and was willing to acknowledge their criticisms as being not unreasonable."[31] Fine's interest in disability perspectives and lived experiences were unusual for genetic counselors in the 1980s and can perhaps be explained, in part, by her unconventional training in the field.

In Omaha, Fine was actively engaged with the parent advocacy group SOFT (Support Organization for Trisomy), which was initially focused on chromosomal disorders—particularly trisomy 13 and 18. These conditions were generally assumed to be fatal very early in life, although with proper care, some people did go on to live for decades. SOFT was founded in 1980 by Kris Holladay, the parent of a child with trisomy 18 in Salt Lake City. Initially, medical geneticist Bruce Buehler cared for Holladay's daughter Kari and then transferred her over to pediatrician John C. Carey (chapter 1) when Buehler moved to Omaha. Buehler brought with him an interest in trisomy 18 and helped to get Fine involved. In 1982, Fine was the lead author, along with Holladay, Carey, and genetic counselor Karen Greendale on a pamphlet titled, *Trisomy 18: A Book for Families*. The book featured many real-life and humanizing photographs and quotes from families affected by this condition and discussed the many challenges that families might face. *Trisomy 18* addressed life support and other interventions immediately after birth and also included discussion of long-term care and support—topics that were often dismissed or overlooked with this and other "lethal" conditions.

Perspectives in Genetic Counseling published a notably critical review of *Trisomy 18* on its front page in 1984. Genetic counselor Dorothy Halperin wrote of the pamphlet,

> There is a gentle suggestion that developmental delay is part of the picture for trisomy 18. The authors do not mention that there are very few long-term survivors or that the retardation can be severe. . . . [O]ne can quickly forget the ominous prognosis that is the general rule for trisomy 18. The exception to the rule, rather than the rule itself, is stressed.

The book, she believed, provided an unrealistic picture of trisomy 18 by focusing on "the very few babies who survive."[32] Genetic counselors, Halperin warned, should think carefully before distributing the pamphlet to their patients.

A few months later, genetic counselor Bonnie Jeanne Baty defended the pamphlet in a letter to the editor, stating,

> I have long felt that our field lacks readable, informative, but humanizing litera-
> ture written for parents about the specific disorder their child has. . . . [T]he only
> thing you can offer [parents] is a series of treatises on cases, autopsy findings,
> mortality and morbidity statistics. . . . [T]here is scarcely a glimpse of the human
> feelings involved in experiencing these events.[33]

The provision of biomedical information, Baty suggested, far outweighed more optimistic accounts of conditions like trisomy 18, including real-life family narratives. Clearly, there was some strong disagreement within ge-netic counseling about what perspectives on disability were most appropri-ate to present. Did patients primarily need biomedical accounts of conditions, which focused on pathology and highlighted the most common anticipated outcomes? Was there also a responsibility for genetic counselors to provide narratives from family experiences outside of the clinic, which offered hope and humanization?

During her career, Fine made the case for broader-based and more opti-mistic views of disabilities in genetic counseling—including conditions that were considered to be "severe." Sadly, Fine's life was cut short in 1998 by a fatal recurrence of breast cancer. Kelly Ormond, who had recently completed her genetic counseling training at Northwestern, took on some of Fine's am-bitions after her passing—including the research partnership with Gill. She also became the director of the Northwestern program.[34] Ormond's subse-quent research with Gill and Kristi Kirschner, which was published in 2000, was some of the earliest scholarship from within the genetic counseling field to actively engage with and promote disability perspectives on the oppres-sive impacts of genetic testing and clinical professionals' attitudes about disabled people.[35]

Gill, Ormond, and Kirschner's important work was by no means the first critique of genetic counseling as it relates to disability. In fact, prominent self-advocates and disability scholars had been targeting genetic counseling for decades, ever since the mid-1980s, when prenatal testing became com-monplace and the Human Genome Project was first being discussed (chap-ter 6).[36] In 1988, the editors of the *Perspectives* newsletter invited critics of genetic counseling to offer disability community viewpoints on the field. Harvard biologist and feminist social activist Ruth Hubbard wrote of genetic counseling,

> To help clients understand the effect that a child with a specific disability may have on their lives, genetic counselors need to understand their particular situation. . . . While genetic counseling programs provide a variety of classroom studies and experiential field work, most are geared toward training in the medical model and do not offer a broad social perspective or incorporate disability training awareness.[37]

Along similar lines, Marsha Saxton, a disability scholar and self-advocate (chapter 6) suggested, "Many clinicians never have the opportunity to see disabled individuals living independently, productively, enjoyably."[38]

Influential training program directors Joan Marks and Seymour Kessler—who were among the field's leading voices for enhancing the psychological counseling skills of genetic counselors—responded to Hubbard's and Saxton's critiques dismissively. They wrote, in a letter to the editors of *Perspectives*, "We see no great merit in giving ideologues an opportunity in the NSGC's own forum to bash the profession and to present it to the outside world and to ourselves in ways that have little or no relationship to reality."[39] Far from engaging with these external observations and concerns, Kessler and Marks rejected these two well-known feminist and disability advocates as outsiders and "ideologues." In fact, the critical arguments of Hubbard and Saxton were relatively mild and focused on concerns that Kessler and Marks had previously highlighted—about the narrowly biomedical focus of genetic counseling training and practice.[40] Nonetheless, Hubbard's and Saxton's suggestions that genetic counseling did harm to disabled people elicited a defensive response rather than reflective engagement by the field's leaders.

In the 1980s and '90s, significant tensions existed between the viewpoints of disability advocates and the perspectives offered by most genetic counseling training programs. Campbell Brasington, a genetic counselor who did her master's training during the late 1980s, recalled, "When I first went into practice . . . I thought as many health professionals did, that the birth of a child with Down syndrome was a devastating and mostly tragic event. . . . My graduate training program did not dissuade me from nor challenge these views."[41] Genetic counseling program directors occasionally criticized overly narrow "medical model" thinking about disability. Some, including Kessler and Marks, pushed for reform through greater attention to counseling skills and other psychosocial aspects of practice. At the same time, outside scholars' suggestions—that the assumptions and approaches of genetic counseling should be critically reexamined because they were overly pessimistic about life with disabilities—were swiftly dismissed as inaccurate.

Advocacy in Genetic Counseling

During the field's first three decades, only a small contingent of genetic counselors actively engaged in promoting and practicing sociopolitical or community-based advocacy related to disability—primarily by joining, leading, or assisting parent support groups outside of the clinical setting. Should disability advocacy, beyond supporting individual patients in the clinic, be part of genetic counselors' professional identity? Many disability advocates who criticized the field in the 1980s and '90s believed that genetic counselors had an important and potentially powerful part to play in reshaping societal perceptions and approaches to disability (chapter 6); whereas, most genetic counselors had much narrower vision of their advocacy role.

Discussions in the genetic counseling profession about practitioners' role as patient advocates were long-standing and widely variable in their views. During the 1970s, medical geneticist Charles Epstein and colleagues expressed concern about references to genetic counselors as patient advocates because, he explained, "the advocacy referred to presumably being directed against the physician." The concept of genetic counselors as clinically based patient advocates troubled physicians who envisioned them becoming a counterweight to their medical authority in determining proper patient care practices. Epstein and other medical geneticists formulated the first official definition of genetic counseling in 1974. It made no reference to advocacy. They defined genetic counseling as a "communication process," which involved assisting patients to understand their genetic diagnosis and risk factors, as well as to respond and adjust to this information in ways that fit with their particular family goals or ethical and religious beliefs.[42]

In 1983, the NSGC board of directors defined genetic counselors as "health professionals with advanced education and experience in the areas of medical genetics and counseling." This definition situated genetic counselors as health care providers, who had a unique mixture of biomedical and psychological expertise. The definition continued, "Genetic counselors also provide supportive counseling to families, serve as patient advocates, and refer families to other support services." While advocacy was included in NSGC's own characterization of genetic counseling, its meaning was relatively narrowly defined in terms of advocating for specific patients. Seemingly, this advocacy would be largely limited to the clinical context, since the same sentence implies that outside referrals would also be made for other support services.[43]

Genetic counselors' identity as advocates was rarely addressed in *Perspectives* during the 1980s and early '90s. However, as pro-life political mobilization grew, some genetic counselors encouraged professional involvement in efforts to protect abortion access and rights. This was a major area of political advocacy for the Society. Though abortion was an increasingly contentious issue in the wider society, NSGC members broadly supported advocacy in this realm (chapter 6).[44] On the other hand, sociopolitical advocacy concerning disability discrimination, stigma, and rights was not promoted by NSGC, even though many members had close personal and professional relationships with disabled people. In 1988, NSGC reported that 95 percent of its members were motivated to become genetic counselors because of a relative or close friend with a genetic disease or birth defect. It was noted that these findings "may account for the high degree of empathy and understanding our profession has for persons with disabilities and our ability to act as patient advocates."[45] Notably, the authors went on to state that, despite their personal experiences, genetic counselors were able to retain their professional commitment to respecting the autonomous reproductive choices of patients. This framing seemed to suggest that it would be *inappropriate* for genetic counselors to engage in practices or advocacy roles that endorsed more positive and accepting views of disability—if this encouraged different outcomes.

Multiple other references to advocacy in the *Perspectives* newsletter focused on the problem of potential conflicts of interest for genetic counselors when they served as advocates. For instance, the challenges inherent in genetic counselors being both "advocates for patients and for science," in the context of their participation or leadership in controlled research trials were noted.[46] Another description of "patient advocacy" in the newsletter involved informing other health professionals about the value of genetic counseling services for their patients—with the goal of ensuring that genetic counseling would remain part of "routine" prenatal care.[47] In this instance, the line between patient advocacy and professional interests was certainly blurred. Clearly, genetic counselors perceived patient advocacy to be part of their pro-

fessional identity, but what this specifically meant for their clinical and societal activities remained poorly defined. Later descriptions of genetic counseling, including one officially developed by an NSGC committee in 2006,
left out the word *advocacy* or any indirect references to it all together.[48]

A notable exception to the above trends was NSGC's first professional
Code of Ethics, adopted in 1992. This document did not specifically mention
advocacy, but it did offer concrete insights on genetic counselors' broader
societal responsibilities. The NSGC Code of Ethics was distinctive among
similar documents produced by other medical and dental professionals in
that it was not structured around considerations of bioethical "principlism,"
which highlighted autonomy, beneficence, nonmaleficence, and justice. This
was particularly striking, given the genetic counseling field's strong commitment to facilitating patient autonomy, against the historical background
of eugenics. Instead, the NSGC chose an "ethics of care" structure, which
focused on the nature of practitioners' relationships with themselves, their
patients, colleagues, and society. In taking this approach, NSGC consciously
aligned its code more closely with those of nursing, counseling, and social
work professions rather than major medical organizations.[49]

Although genetic counseling training and practice, like much of medicine, was strongly oriented around individual relationships and responsibilities to patients, the NSGC Code of Ethics noted the need for a broader
positive role in society. The Code's authors wrote, "Many forms of unjust
discrimination exist in our society. . . . As individuals, and as professionals,
genetic counselors should maintain an acute awareness of discriminatory
practices, with the goal of minimizing such practices in our society."[50] A further explication of genetic counselors' identity as proponents of social change
under the Code of Ethics encouraged practitioners to be reliable sources of
information for policymakers and the public. It also highlighted helping to
eliminate discrimination, citing many forms such as race, gender, and age—
but not disability.[51]

In line with these goals, NSGC's first committee on diversity among genetic counselors was formed in 1993. Its members argued that increasing the
diversity of the field's practitioners was an important strategy for addressing societal discrimination and improving clinical services for marginalized
populations. The committee began a multidecade effort to increase diversity
among genetic counselors—calling for improved representation by race, ethnicity, cultural heritage, gender, *and* disability. Over the next 25 years, NSGC

considered the potential impacts of having greater professional diversity around various social identities, but the specific value of attracting more disabled genetic counselors was left notably unexplored.[52] Disability often made the list of diverse social identities, but it clearly was not a primary target for change.

Like practitioners of other marginalized social identities, disabled genetic counselors can bring greater cultural and experiential diversity to the field. They may speak directly to the societal discrimination that disabled people face in the clinic and the wider world, and about various perspectives from within disability communities about how to counter such oppression. As part of this, disabled genetic counselors would also be likely to introduce more critical perspectives on biomedical conceptions of disability and genetic counselors' role in prenatal testing and selective abortion—issues that the field has remained resistant to addressing.

Notably, revisions to the NSGC Code of Ethics in 2017 narrowed genetic counselors' purview to preventing only "genetic discrimination," which targeted individual markers of genetic "risk." The authors also removed language calling for practitioners to "participate in activities necessary to bring about socially responsible change," because this expectation "was not sufficiently specific to genetics."[53] These revisions further distanced genetic counseling from having a broad-based role in fighting discrimination based on social identity. For advocates who hoped to see NSGC place a greater emphasis on countering societal disability discrimination, by way of professional inclusion and political advocacy, such changes were in the wrong direction.

The "Counseling" Role

The original NSGC Code of Ethics and various targeted efforts to enhance the field's diversity were representative of genetic counselors' greater reflection and interrogation of their professional identity and role in the 1990s. By this time, genetic counseling had become a well-established field, and its practioners' knowledge and skills were sought after—particularly in the context of the Human Genome Project and the many social and ethical concerns associated with it.[54] The prevalence of genetic markers for clinical conditions was increasing rapidly, as were tests developed to detect them. Amid this, genetic counselors successfully positioned themselves as experts on clinically relevant genetic markers who possessed on-the-ground understanding of consumer concerns and uptake.

In 1993, the genetic counseling field took a major step forward in establishing its own professional autonomy by breaking away from physician medical geneticists to found the American Board of Genetic Counseling, an independent accrediting body. Proponents of this move argued, "Times and circumstances have changed. Genetic counselors have grown in maturity, experience, respect, and number. . . . [W]e have developed guidelines for continuing education programs and established a presence in the community at large."[55] As the field gained respect and independence among clinical professionals, some of its practitioners began to more vigorously reconsider and challenge certain long-standing elements of its practices and goals.

The genetic counseling profession was universally committed to: (1) providing accessible and accurate genetic knowledge to patients; and (2) the ideal of facilitating informed and autonomous choices about genetic testing and what to do with results. These two goals were unavoidably interrelated. Master's level genetic counselors were constantly mindful of the need to distance their field from its historical eugenic roots in "improving" the gene pool, as well as to avoid the potential for intentional societal manipulation by way of reproductive choices. To achieve this, genetic counseling had embraced the principle of "nondirective" practice during the 1970s—in which practitioners consciously avoided allowing their own assumptions and beliefs from influencing patient decision-making.[56] By the late 1990s, many genetic counselors had concluded that nondirective approaches were neither possible—because a practitioner's assumptions and biases always influenced their counseling—nor in the best interests of patients, who benefited from, or desired to hear, their counselor's own perspectives. This realization was widely viewed by genetic counselors as a positive step forward for their field, but it left the profession without a unifying model of how to best achieve its dual goals of information provision and facilitating autonomous choice.[57] The best path forward was a matter of diverse opinions and debate. A major focus of this discussion during the 1990s and 2000s was on the meaning and relative importance of the *genetic* and *counseling* components of practice.

Late twentieth-century physicians often valued genetic counselors for their empathy and communication skills. Ralph Amato, a medical geneticist, recounted that genetic counselors were often much better than physicians at using descriptive language that patients could comprehend and more concerned with making sure that patients did understand. Pediatrician John C. Carey recalled that, as a medical genetics fellow, he learned a lot more from genetic counselors about how to talk to patients and families than he ever had in medical school. Genetic counselors set a high bar for thoughtful and reflective communication, which Carey felt pressure to achieve.[58]

Many leaders in the genetic counseling field also viewed compassionate and accessible communication as the primary goal of the "counseling" component of practice. As Virginia Corson, an early NSGC president, put it, "What we talk about with families is a lot of science, but how we talk about it is the counseling." Brenda Finucane, who served as NSGC president in 2012, posited,

> I bet if the field was invented today, "counseling" would not be part of the terminology. We all value the counseling, because we know how important it is to disclose the information in the appropriate way, but I think that the "counseling" word leads to the public misconception that genetic counseling is a psychology field, when in fact it is a very technical, scientific field.[59]

Indeed, many turn-of-the-century genetic counselors believed that the helpful and conscientious provision of biomedical information was their primary purpose and the main reason why physicians and patients valued their expertise. Bonnie LeRoy, a program director and previous NSGC president noted, "The truth is the people who come into our clinics primarily come for information. Counseling skills are a vehicle for communicating that information in a manner that people can understand and use. Unlike in counseling psychology, we don't want to change anyone's behavior, we just want to help them understand what happened."[60]

A smaller contingent of genetic counselors viewed the "counseling" aspect of their practice as having goals that stretched well beyond the provision of information. Barbara Biesecker, a former training program director and NSGC president, suggested,

> I think genetic counselors ended up over time really falling back on giving people information, especially as we learned more, and had more to tell people. And they don't do the counseling. . . . The information cannot define who we are. There are always going to be better ways for people to get the information, but how does it relate to a patient's personal values, interests, and needs?[61]

For these practitioners, communication of genetic information was not the primary goal of their interactions with patients. Dynamic and in-depth counseling was also an important professional ambition. In fact, this was the part of genetic counseling they were most passionate about and that they be-lieved made the field so unique. As genetic counselor Ellyn Farrelly noted, "The truth is people can look up online all of their options for testing. I really like to spend the time I have with the patient helping them move to a new place and a deeper understanding."[62]

During the mid-1990s, a few genetic counselors prominently questioned the balance of science and counseling in their field. Writing in the *Perspectives* newsletter, two genetic counselors drew attention to the preponderance of recent genetic counseling master's theses that focused on basic science rather than on counseling practices. They noted that in 1994, five of six student theses from the University of Cincinnati training program were clearly in the former category. The program's director, Nancy Steinberg Warren, soon expressed her discontent with this comment, calling it "neither supportive or encouraging." She responded, "Isn't having understanding of basic science a major part of genetic counseling?" Betty Gettig, another training program director, also pointed out the reality that opportunities and financial support for students were more prevalent in the basic sciences. Further, she argued that counseling skills were better learned through clinical training anyway rather than in master's thesis research.[63] Over the next three years, the titles of student theses from various training programs were regularly printed in the *Perspectives* newsletter, further revealing that biomedical topics consistently outnumbered projects on psychosocial and counseling issues by a large margin.

The academic autonomy and prestige of postwar clinical professions were often tied to having a distinctive base of research and theory (chapter 5). Thus, a lack of research specifically related to genetic counseling theory and practice from within the field was quite concerning. The founding of the *Journal of Genetic Counseling* in 1992, which provided a specific forum for peer-reviewed discipline-specific research, was an important first step in addressing this problem. Nonetheless, decades later many of the genetic counselors I interviewed specifically described their active commitment to staying up-to-date on cutting edge biomedical research, but acknowledged only passive engagement with the latest "counseling" related research, methods, and practice. They described learning about these topics primarily through attending occasional sessions at the NSGC annual conference rather than by seeking out new academic literature.

Late twentieth-century genetic counselors' clinical engagement with patients was also heavily focused on biomedical factors and considerations. Over many years, bioethicist Dorothy Wertz interviewed genetic counseling patients to assess which topics were addressed in their sessions. In 1998, she reported that psychosocial topics—such as costs, family resources, societal impacts, and the effects of having a disabled child on a family's well-being and employment—were only discussed in 2–4 percent of sessions and mentioned 4–8 percent of the time. This ratio was little changed from her analysis a decade earlier. By comparison, the reasons why a disorder occurred, treatment options, and genetic testing were discussed much more frequently. After Wertz presented her findings at the NSGC annual conference in 1998, an article in *Perspectives* noted, "The audience reacted strongly with many pointing out that topics covered depended largely on individual circumstances."[64] Idiosyncratic cases aside, Wertz's results clearly showed that genetic counseling conversations were overwhelmingly focused on biomedical considerations.

Along similar lines, in 1993 sociologist James Sorenson dismissed the claim, put forth by former University of California, Berkeley program director Seymour Kessler, that genetic counseling had undergone a "paradigm shift" since the 1970s toward a greater focus on psychological counseling. While Sorenson acknowledged that some genetic counseling master's programs had attempted to increase the level of counseling training they provided, he argued, "genetic counseling has been, and remains in large part misnamed. . . . I think the weight of evidence suggests that the label of 'genetic consult' more aptly describes what usually transpires in 'genetic counseling.'"[65] Soreson's analysis closely lines up with Finucane's suggestion that practitioners would be named something different if the field were invented in 2018—perhaps "genetics specialists."[66] Although a small contingent of genetic counselors strongly believed that the field should expand its reach beyond a primary commitment to providing accurate and accessible biomedical information, few practitioners appeared to have the desire, or the training necessary, to move in this direction.

In the late 1990s, NSGC tacitly moved to downplay the field's association with active psychosocial counseling. Seeking to further situate the discipline as a health care profession with unique genetics expertise, NSGC launched a marketing campaign titled GeneAMP (Applied Marketing Project). The name alone made clear which aspects of "genetic counseling" were to be high-lighted. NSGC's "One Voice, One Message" marketing team introduced the acronym CARE to describe genetic counselors' primary roles: "**C**an interpret complex family histories and genetic test results. . . . **A**ccess and provide up-to-date information. **R**eview and select the most appropriate quality, cost effective care. **E**ducate families and facilitate decision making."[67]

Immediate pushback came from a select group of genetic counselors, in-cluding Biesecker and Judith Benkendorf, who had led NSGC's 1992 Code of Ethics Committee. They argued that the NSGC marketing campaign's focus "omits, perhaps, our most important area of expertise, that of counseling. . . . [I]t is our counseling skills that will sustain our professional growth." While they acknowledged that counseling was often less well compensated by man-aged health care insurance providers compared to genetics expertise, they encouraged NSGC to be a leader in defining the future of the genetic coun-seling field rather than promoting the profession in ways that "merely re-spond to economic pressures and the ideas of others."[68]

In response, members of NSGC's marketing team—who were themselves genetic counselors—noted that they had conducted a survey of genetic coun-selors who worked in managed health care organizations and found that "psychosocial aspects of counseling all scored predominantly at the 'not important' level." Thus, since the value of counseling was not recognized by managed care providers, the team had decided to leave it out of their mar-keting message. They suggested, however, that while the word was absent, the concept of counseling was still "sewn throughout the message. How can we educate families and facilitate decision-making without calling upon the most basic counseling skills?"[69] This argument mirrored the long-standing perspective of many genetic counseling training program directors, who be-lieved that the counseling component of practice was mostly about deliver-ing accessible and empathetic biomedical information. NSGC's One Voice, One Message marketing team reasonably assumed that, to achieve these goals, genetic counselors did not need more sophisticated counseling skills.

Most genetic counselors believed that both genetics expertise *and* coun-seling, whatever the term implied, were fundamental parts of their profes-sional role and identity. From a training and continuing education perspec-tive, maintaining an adequate balance between these two areas was difficult, due to the ceaseless flow of new genetic knowledge and testing options about which genetic counselors felt they needed to be proficient. This problem was particularly acute because the field's professional training programs lasted just two years. With the constant need to include new and increasingly complex biomedical knowledge, program directors lamented how difficult it was to add, or even retain, psychosocial and counseling components of their curricula. Nonetheless, following the lead of Joan Marks's early efforts to reshape training at Sarah Lawrence, many genetic counseling programs found ways to adopt their own unique emphases.

Innovative Training Programs and Directors

By 1999, there were 25 genetic counseling master's programs in the United States. Beyond the content required by the American Board of Medical Genetics, these programs adopted various specialized interests and approaches. A small number chose to invest in disability-related perspectives, experiences, and community engagement. Most of these innovative programs were founded in the 1990s, and a few identified disability as a central focus from the outset. In addition to the training program at Northwestern University I discussed previously in this chapter and one at Brandeis University (chapter 6), genetic counseling master's programs at the University of California (UC), Berkeley and at Johns Hopkins University/National Institutes of Health (JHU/NIH) stood out for their commitment to enhanced training in counseling, community engagement, and disability perspectives during the 1990s.

The UC Berkeley training program, founded in 1973, was one of the field's oldest and longest running before it closed in 2004. During these years, the program stood out for requiring its students to participate in community-based, nongenetic "clinical" experiences for 12–16 hours each week during their first year. The locations included social service agencies, disability support centers, and public schools. Margie Goldstein, who graduated from the program in 1981 and later returned as codirector, noted that UC Berkeley wanted its students to know more about the social identities, challenges, and experiences of people in the wider community before they learned about patients in a biomedical setting. As part of this, students attended a weekly class in which they discussed and processed their experiences, including how the community supported and failed people across the life span. Goldstein recalled that these experiences were "hugely influential" for her as a student and "maybe the single most important contribution that the Berkeley program made to [training in] the genetic counseling field."[70] From the very beginning, of their time at Berkeley, students were encouraged and empowered to think about their patients in a broader social context and to be aware and involved in community advocacy. This commitment and orientation truly set the Berkeley program apart from its peers.

Seymour Kessler, who directed the UC Berkeley genetic counseling program from 1977 to 1985, had a major hand in shaping its unique reputation as a training program that emphasized enhanced counseling practices. Kessler held a PhD in genetics and earned a second PhD in social and clinical psychology from the Wright Institute in Berkeley. He was strongly committed to client-centered counseling, as well as training genetic counselors to steadfastly and efficiently help their patients to work through extremely difficult and time-sensitive decisions. As part of this, Kessler pushed for training and research methods that incorporated the critical analysis of audio transcripts from genetic counseling sessions. He believed that this was the only way to accurately assess counselors' effectiveness. These approaches shocked many genetic counselors, who felt Kessler was disregarding patient *and* counselor privacy. Unfazed, Kessler displayed his own counseling transcripts at NSGC conferences. In one, he very directly told a pregnant client in a crisis situation that she needed to stop crying so that they could get started on the difficult decision-making task ahead of them. While Kessler's techniques troubled some practitioners, he was a very influential mentor for a small contingent, who privileged in-depth counseling skills.[71]

Jon Weil later led the Berkeley program after Kessler had retired. Weil similarly held a PhD in genetics and had acquired a second doctorate in social and clinical psychology from the Wright Institute. During the 1990s, Weil kept up UC Berkeley's strong focus on counseling skills and community engagements—a set of commitments that became increasingly difficult to maintain as new molecular techniques and gene mapping continuously revolutionized and expanded genetic testing. Notably, Weil drew on and benefited from the significant efforts of genetic counselor Beth Crawford, who had served for four years as interim program director. They helped to introduce a greater focus on multicultural and disability perspectives and issues, including examinations of differing ethnic groups' views of genetic counseling. As part of this, disability self-advocates and scholars, including Marsha Saxton were invited to lead classes.[72]

Weil was strongly influenced by sociologists Troy Duster and Diane Beeson, as well as disability scholar and self-advocate Adrienne Asch (chapters

1 and 6), as he began to formulate his own perspectives on the practice of genetic counseling. In 2000, he published *Psychosocial Genetic Counseling*, a textbook focusing on counseling techniques. As someone who entered genetic counseling in his mid-career and was never formally trained in a master's program, Weil viewed himself as a relative outsider. He brought a distinctive intellectual perspective to the field and sought to introduce more sociological viewpoints—in particular through his textbook's final chapter. He noted, "I felt very strongly about the last chapter in my book. The first seven chapters were just establishing my credentials to write what I did in the last chapter."[73]

Weil's closing chapter drew on social science research analyzing the various reasons why patients resisted genetic testing. Along with religious beliefs and "romantic" considerations—the desire to have whatever child comes from a specific partnership—this scholarship highlighted the ways in which experiential knowledge of disability led people to thoughtfully resist prenatal genetic testing. In direct contrast, many genetic counselors were taught to presume that the rejection of genetic testing, especially in the absence of religious considerations, suggested emotional, psychodynamically complex, or ill-informed decision-making. Weil argued that turning down prenatal testing based on experiences with disability was rational, but that genetic counselors and their patients often lacked a common language for articulating and justifying this reasoning.[74] He also pointed to research showing that patients' more critical beliefs about genetic testing often went unexpressed and unexplored when genetic counselors emphasized clinical and technical considerations. Weil noted that genetic counselors needed to possess a strong desire to dig deeper to uncover the patients' perspectives and values. Absent a push from genetic counselors to engage further, conversations were more likely to remain abstractly biomedical.[75]

Psychosocial Genetic Counseling seriously and thoroughly engaged with the disability rights movement and "social model" critiques and perspectives. Weil highlighted Saxton's and Asch's critiques of negative and narrowly biomedical views of disability (chapters 1 and 6), arguing that "continuing and increasing contacts among genetic counselors, individuals with disabilities, and disability rights activists are of great importance" because self-advocates brought to the discipline important, alternative views of life and experiences with a disability.[76] He further suggested that, whether or not the field wanted to be associated with an identity as sociopolitical advocates, genetic counselors' involvement in prenatal testing and selective abortion unavoidably made them agents of social change. He hoped that greater engagement with critical perspectives on prenatal genetic diagnosis and counseling would lead to "increased awareness and motivation to advocate for change."[77] Undoubtedly, Weil's integration of disability perspectives had a significant influence on UC Berkeley students and other genetic counselors. Decades after his book's publication, though, he remained uncertain about its impact on the field's views of disability. Despite this, Weil did know that Asch was heartened by his career trajectory—from laboratory scientist, to genetic counselor, to strong disability advocate.[78]

Barbara Biesecker at JHU / NIH was another important figure within genetic counseling who eventually began to seriously engage with disability perspectives in her publications. The JHU / NIH genetic counseling master's program was founded by Biesecker, Don Hadley, and Barbara Bernhardt in 1996. Biesecker had been strongly influenced by Kessler as an early career genetic counselor and promoted the program as emphasizing advanced counseling skills.[79] The JHU / NIH program was unique in extending an extra six months beyond the usual two-year time line, which allowed more room for additional psychosocially oriented courses, along with the required heavy focus on biomedical content and clinical rotations. Trainees at JHU / NIH attended frequent seminars featuring patient advocates and perspectives and received weekly supervision where a faculty mentor helped each student reflect on their own counseling-related responses, emotions, and experiences. Such oversight and support was standard practice in mental health fields. Biesecker had always found it concerning that genetic counseling training programs did not include supervision.[80]

During the late 1990s and early 2000s, Biesecker and some of her colleagues in the JHU / NIH program were outspoken proponents of disability critiques and perspectives on genetic counseling. Biesecker had gotten to know Asch and Saxton through various meetings that brought together clinicians, ethicists, and disability advocates (chapter 6). In 2000, Biesecker and current trainee Lori Hamby wrote,

> Families would be best served by being encouraged to examine these [disability] issues throughout their lifetimes. Genetic professionals can aid in such encouragement. However, people will not truly be prepared for considering the relevant issues during genetic counseling until society as a whole begins to embrace

these same topics. . . . [W]e propose that *all* members of our society would benefit from a broad, public examination of how we do—and should—understand
"normal" and "valuable" (emphasis in original).[81]

Biesecker and Hamby argued that genetic counselors needed to be aware of
their own biases about disability and recognize that many of their clients
were strongly influenced by society's overly pessimistic views as well. Rather
than accepting this as unavoidable, Biesecker and Hamby envisioned societal programs that could alter these trends and an active role for genetic
counselors in changing perceptions.

The JHU / NIH program incorporated multiple nonclinical interactions
with disabled people. Students did a project with a disability support group,
took a semester-long course on disability perspectives, and got to know disabled people and their families outside of the clinic. As a student, Hamby
volunteered at a Muscular Dystrophy Association overnight camp, which provided her with significant extraclinical and personal experience and awareness of children with neuromuscular conditions. She continued to work at
the camp for over a decade, built strong connections with families and disability advocates in the area, and eventually specialized in counseling and
research related to neuromuscular disabilities. When Biesecker stepped down
as director of the JHU / NIH program in 2017, Lori Hamby Erby took over the
position, with the intention of maintaining Biesecker's vision and priorities
for training genetic counselors.[82]

Meanwhile, UC Berkeley discontinued its genetic counseling master's
program in 2004 soon after Weil retired. The program had no lack of students, applicants, or respect in the field. Rather, the UC Berkeley School of
Public Health chose not to house the program any longer, and no new location in the UC system was immediately identified. Given its long-standing
and unique investment in community engagement, the closing of UC Berkeley's training program was a significant loss to the field. Years later, Goldstein founded a new program at California State University Stanislaus, which
was partly modeled on the UC Berkeley program.[83]

Late twentieth-century genetic counseling was a highly biomedical and
primarily clinically based profession. Training programs at Northwestern,
JHU / NIH, UC Berkeley, and Brandeis (chapter 6) stood out for adding valuable new perspectives. Their directors uniquely placed community-based
training, advanced counseling techniques, and disability advocacy and aware-

ness at the forefront of the programs' ambitions and identity. While they began as outliers in the profession, over time these four programs became models for how genetic counseling could differently address training on disability and sociopolitical advocacy. Importantly, after 2000 these elements and approaches were more widely adopted by other programs in the field.

Conclusions

Broadly speaking, postwar genetic counselors were indifferent to calls from a small but vocal minority of their colleagues for the field to further develop its counseling role beyond the accessible and empathetic provision of biomedical information. Most genetic counselors were also hesitant to engage in social and political advocacy outside of the clinical context—and in some prominent venues were highly dismissive toward critical disability perspectives on the discipline and its role in prenatal testing. NSGC, for its part, tended to highlight an identity for genetic counselors as biomedical experts and roles as clinically based educators as advocates for individual patients and families. These were reasonable points of emphasis, especially since practitioners' role and identity as skilled genetic communicators and consultants helped to establish and maintain the field's value and prestige relative to other clinical professions.

Postwar genetic counselors frequently overlooked or resisted adopting more positive and inclusive narratives of disability and generally chose not to engage in clinical or community-based activities that would help implement more optimistic and accepting perspectives on life with disabilities among their patients, colleagues, and the general public. These stances had the effect of perpetuating more pessimistic and pathological viewpoints on disability—as a "risk" to be avoided rather than as a socially imposed status or a valued form of diversity. Amid this, some genetic counseling training directors positioned their programs to counter narrow and negative views of disability through greater engagement and awareness of disability experiences and scholarly perspectives. Still, though, as I describe further in chapter 6, many other influential leaders in the field chose to double down on a professional role and identity in facilitating and protecting patients' reproductive choice, while offering primarily biomedical views of disability.

Late twentieth-century genetic counseling was a demographically and intellectually homogeneous field.[84] About 95 percent of genetic counselors were white women, and most came from middle-class backgrounds with undergraduate degrees in biology or psychology. I believe it is significant that many of the "outlier" training programs highlighted in this chapter were founded or strongly influenced by directors who did not hold master's degrees in genetic counseling. Perhaps, not surprisingly, practitioners who entered genetic counseling through nontraditional pathways were more likely to campaign for the field to move in new directions. While the field's identity and ambitions were very much up for grabs initially, once prenatal testing came to dominate its clinical practices, very few genetic counselors were open to reimagining their primary roles and sociopolitical commitments. Notably, those who did call for significant changes in approaching disability were often strongly influenced by self-advocates, who played a leading role in encouraging genetic counselors and other clinicians to reconsider their priorities.

Synthesis and Next Steps

My first three chapters offer a broad history of clinical psychology, pediatrics, and genetic counseling and their postwar engagement with disability advocacy and perspectives. While outright pessimism toward the prospects of disabled people declined in each field over time, these disciplines maintained consistent professional identities, roles, and markers of prestige that encouraged continued resistance to new disability narratives. Clinical psychologists emphasized their professional role in training patients to adjust to and cope with disabilities—rather than incorporating a broader social systems view on the sources of disability experiences and stigma. Pediatricians highlighted an identity as uniquely qualified team leaders and community-based care coordinators—even as their conception and focus on disabilities remained primarily medical, and their engagement with institutions beyond the clinic was quite limited.

Genetic counselors identified with the role of patient educators and a primary identity as genetics experts. Very few genetic counselors adopted a parallel identity as advocates for more positive, inclusive, and sociopolitical perspectives on disability. All three fields primarily focused on individual-level, clinically or biomedically based research and advocacy, despite the efforts of many disability advocates to encourage more sociopolitical perspectives. As part of this, each discipline showed limited or negligible interest in addressing disability discrimination within their own professional domain, especially in terms of attracting more disabled people to their training programs and supporting them throughout their education and careers.

Over the next three chapters, I examine a number of specific case studies within each clinical field. These more isolated events took place within the broader history and professional considerations described in the first three chapters. Targeted case studies offer opportunities to analyze particular instances in which concerns about professional identity, role, and prestige informed reluctant and resistant responses to new, more positive, inclusive, and sociopolitically oriented perspectives and approaches to disability. I begin in chapters 4 and 5 by turning to specific debates in late twentieth-century clinical psychology and pediatrics about appropriate understandings and engagement with disability and how these discussions were informed by various professional, social, and political contexts involving science, social advocacy, and career advancement.

In chapter 6, I focus specifically on the critiques of disability scholars, self-advocates, and organizations of genetic counselors' role in facilitating prenatal diagnosis and selective abortion. As in other chapters, particular attention is given to how disability advocates directly—and often through personal relationships—influenced the viewpoints and narratives of clinical professionals. Examining genetic counselors' investments in and approaches to prenatal testing offers opportunities to more extensively consider the perceptions and status of the field within wider social and clinical contexts, as well as the ways in which genetic counselors' relationships with disability self-advocates were influenced by broader political contexts in recent US history.

4

Advocacy before Evidence?

Disability Controversies in Clinical Psychology

In December 1986, the board of directors of the American Association on Mental Deficiency (AAMD) approved a new position statement op-
posing the continued use of "aversive therapies." These interventions involved physical and psychological punishment, including forced exposure
to unpleasant tastes or smells, electroshocks, pinching, and humiliation.
Some clinical psychologists had been using aversives since the mid-1960s to
modify or reduce certain behaviors in autistic people and individuals with
intellectual disabilities that they considered to be unusual, disruptive, self-
injurious, or otherwise dangerous.[1] AAMD condemned the use of aversives
in these patient populations and urged immediate elimination of interventions causing obvious signs of physical pain, potential physical side effects,
or dehumanization. The board of directors also encouraged ongoing research
into alternative, nonpunishment approaches.[2]

This had not been the Association's first position statement on aversives. A decade earlier, AAMD addressed the use of painful interventions
meant to modify behavior by calling for informed consent, frequent reviews
of effectiveness, systems for minimizing risk, and review bodies to consider
long-term consequences associated with "exposure to risk, pain, or infringe-
ment of dignity."[3] Their earlier statement in no way condemned aversives.
Rather, it accepted the existence of and need for these interventions, arguing only for improved oversight.

As I describe throughout this chapter, the significant differences between the 1975 and 1986 AAMD statements on aversive therapies reflected
larger philosophical shifts within the Association, as well as other disability-
focused clinical professional groups, during the late twentieth century. Many

clinical practitioners had begun turning away from viewing aversives as necessary, short-term interventions for extreme cases of destructive or self-injurious behavior and instead started to perceive these approaches as unacceptably dehumanizing in all circumstances. These changing views on aversives also paralleled ongoing reassessments and debates among clinical psychologists about institutionalization (chapter 1). While some clinical practitioners saw residential institutions as harmful and dehumanizing locations that needed to be closed entirely and immediately, others had vested professional interests in institutions and argued that they were necessary and beneficial for certain individuals and families. Along similar lines, even as opposition to aversives grew in the 1980s, calls to ban them entirely remained controversial.

AAMD had experienced previous periods of transition. Founded in 1876 as the Association of Medical Officers of American Institutions for Idiotic and Feebleminded persons, throughout much of its first century, the organization was primarily a professional home for the physician administrators of residential institutions.[4] During the 1960s, as professional engagement and jurisdiction over intellectual and developmental disabilities began to shift, a number of reform-minded pediatricians, including Richard Koch, Robert Kugel, and Margaret Giannini (chapter 2), took up leadership positions in AAMD. By the 1980s, psychologists and special educators increasingly dominated the organization. They pushed through various long sought-after changes, including a new name in 1987—the American Association on Mental Retardation (AAMR), which (at the time) they viewed as less offensive. By the mid-2000s, most of the Association's original membership base of physician administrators of residential institutions had decamped to a new organization. This once again facilitated a name change, in 2007, to the American Association on Intellectual and Developmental Disabilities (AAIDD).[5]

Meanwhile, many psychologists who specialized in intellectual and developmental disabilities felt increasingly marginalized in AAMR and gravitated instead to Division 33 of the American Psychological Association (APA). Psychologist Thomas McCulloch, who worked in a residential institution conducting experimental primate and clinical research on intellectual disabilities, played a central role in founding Division 33 during the early 1970s. Division 33 members often had a strong scientific identity and focused on individual-level assessments and interventions. Many were experimental and behaviorist researchers who held the theories of B. F. Skinner in high regard. Some Division 33 psychologists, including O. Ivar Lovaas and Donald M. Baer, were major contributors to the field of Applied Behavior Analysis (ABA), which drew from Skinnerian behaviorist theories. ABA used positive reinforcement and negative stimuli—like painful aversives—to achieve behavior modification in individuals with intellectual and developmental disabilities, particularly for children that engaged in self-injurious behaviors.[6]

As in AAMR the leaders of APA Division 33 were also deeply invested in multiple ideological battles related to intellectual and developmental disabilities during the late twentieth century. In his 1999 historical account of Division 33, psychologist Donald Routh described four major accomplishments during the group's first 25 years. Along with efforts to increase federal dollars for disability research, Routh identified as significant Division 33's activities in: (1) supporting the continued need for aversives; (2) criticizing AAMR's new classification scheme for mental retardation; and (3) challenging the scientific validity of facilitated communication.[7]

In this chapter, I examine all three of these controversial issues as they related to clinical psychology and evolving conceptions of disability. For psychologists, each was both novel and divisive because it involved the efforts by some of their own colleagues—along with special educators—to move away from describing and addressing intellectual and developmental disabilities primarily at the level of individual deficits and interventions. Proponents of these new directions sought to reduce stigma and dehumanization, while increasing optimistic narratives and societal support for disabled people. In doing so, special educators and some psychologists challenged long-standing presumptions and methodologies associated with measuring, assessing, and treating people with intellectual and developmental disabilities and behavioral differences. Many Division 33 members viewed such novel approaches as threatening to their professional expertise and jurisdiction. As part of this, they argued that these new directions lacked support from controlled, empirical studies or directly contradicted existing scientific knowledge.

Meanwhile, professionals who had family members with intellectual and developmental disabilities were important leaders in various efforts to reform psychological approaches and encourage more positive, inclusive, and sociopolitical perspectives on disability, despite significant reluctance and criticism from some of their psychologist colleagues. Special educators also played a significant role in promoting more optimistic, accepting, and environmentally oriented views of disabled people. In some instances, psychologists collaborated with special educators, while in others—particularly around facilitated communication—psychologists were much more resolutely opposed to educators' efforts. As I show, central to these differing perspectives were questions posed by psychologists about whether robust, blinded, and reproducible experimental methods supported new views and approaches.

During the late twentieth century, some psychologists rethought and challenged the universal value and predominance of certain forms of scientific expertise, methodologies, and ways of knowing related to intellectual and developmental disabilities. Amid this, novel perspectives on disabled people led to significant professional conflict and tribalism, which continued into the 2000s. In this chapter, I argue that many clinical psychologists resisted the adoption of more positive, inclusive, and sociopolitically oriented disability perspectives because these views threatened the preeminence of their favored scientific theories and measures, as well as their expertise in individual-level clinical assessment and interventions. Even though newer approaches were intended to enhance the perceived potential and reduce the stigma associated with their patients, these clinical psychologists viewed them as scientifically invalid and rooted in "biased" epistemologies—privileging hope, humanism, and sociopolitical conceptions of disability—that drew upon a different set of values from rigorous empirical analysis.

The Push to Eliminate Aversives

In 1981, the executive board of the Association for the Severely Handicapped (TASH) became the first major professional and advocacy organization to approve a resolution calling for the immediate cessation of using aversive procedures for behavior modification in people with developmental disabilities. TASH was founded six years earlier by a small group of educators and psychologists who had met informally at AAMD's annual conference and agreed that existing organizations were overly focused on professional concerns rather than on political advocacy for people with "severe" disabilities. Around the same time, the US federal government passed PL 94-142, the Education for All Handicapped Children Act, which mandated access to free and developmentally appropriate public education for all children in their own community (chapter 2). TASH took a leading role in helping the US Department of Education enact the provisions of this law. As part of this, the group advocated for continued deinstitutionalization and for the full and equal societal inclusion of disabled people.[8]

TASH's resolution on aversives highlighted the importance of access to effective treatment, education, and habilitative services, as well as, "the equally important right to freedom from harm," including signs of pain, physical side effects, and dehumanization.[9] The document was initially controversial within TASH.[10] While the group focused on sociopolitical advocacy, its membership was made up largely of professionals, some of who were sympathetic to the argument that aversive procedures were useful or necessary in some cases. As TASH cofounder and psychologist Wayne Sailor later put it, "Throughout its history, TASH has undergone numerous stresses and strains having largely to do with the desire on the part of [disability] self-advocates to have TASH be their organization as its primary mission, versus the researchers, trainers, and other, primarily university based, persons who wanted to keep TASH as a scientifically oriented forum for credible public policy."[11] Opposition to aversives fit with TASH's advocacy goals. For clinical professionals, though, there was little empirical evidence—about efficacy, side effects, or viable alternatives—that could be pointed to in support of the ban.

Clinical psychologists did not pay much attention to TASH's resolution on aversives. TASH was still a fledgling upstart and did not have the established legitimacy and authority of the much older and larger AAMD. Five years later, however, AAMD's position statement calling for the elimination of aversive therapies immediately generated vigorous responses and intense debates. Clinical psychologists who believed that aversives needed to be available for certain patients and situations spoke up in opposition to AAMD's significant shift. In a letter to AAMD's *News and Notes* professional newsletter, clinical psychologist and Division 33 member Johnny L. Matson expressed serious concerns that AAMD's position would lead to legislation banning the use of aversives. As he put it, the statement could set up "the Orwellian specter of government rather than professionals regulating treatments."[12] Matson was concerned about maintaining his field's established expert identity and jurisdiction in the area of behavioral interventions for people with developmental disabilities.[13] He argued that clinical psychologists who used aversives were the professionals best positioned to determine their value for patients.

AAMD's executive board certainly understood that their new position on aversives would anger many clinical psychologists—who comprised a large portion of the Association's membership. Why then did AAMD leaders move so suddenly and stringently to oppose aversives? The 1980s was a time of significant change at AAMD, as it continued to move away from a long-standing role as the primary professional organization for physician administrators of residential institutions. AAMD became more involved in socio-political advocacy and restructured its membership categories "to invite and encourage active participation by direct care personnel, paraprofessionals, and consumers."[14] In 1987, AAMD also changed its name to the more progressive—for the time—American Association on Mental Retardation.

Lawyer and special education professor H. Rutherford Turnbull III was a major driving force behind these changes. Turnbull was also a family advocate. His teenage son Jay had significant developmental disabilities. During his 1985–86 term as AAMD president, Turnbull pushed for an ongoing shift in focus toward advocacy and away from professional concerns. He also expressed strong support for developing AAMD's more critical stance on aversive procedures.[15] Jay was an advocate as well—he later worked for two decades at Kansas University's Beach Center on Disability, contributing to its efforts to enhance opportunities for people with disabilities.[16]

Meanwhile, many rank-and-file AAMD members, especially those in the psychology division, argued that the executive board's position statement on aversives needed to be revisited.[17] Clinical psychologist Joseph B. Keys noted that "the Association did not submit the proposal to the membership, or request comments and concerns. . . . [It] has not encouraged thoughtful and technically sophisticated review and exchange of information regarding the issue of aversive therapy."[18] Other opponents of AAMD's new position suggested that the call to eliminate aversives was premature given the lack of alternative options. As clinical psychologist Thomas Linscheid put it, "Despite the fervent hope that someday, well-researched positive alternatives will be available to treat any and all severe behavioral problems, at present this is not a reality. For organizations to adopt categorically anti-aversive positions and to advocate for anti-aversive legislation based on a hope is a disservice to individuals with severe behavior disorders."[19] Indeed, even the strongest opponents of aversives acknowledged that little work had been done on developing and assessing alternatives.[20] AAMD had called for more efforts in this area, but many clinical psychologists believed that the loss of aversive options would harm some patients.

Eventually, an AAMR task force comprising psychologists, special educators, and other specialists was established to revisit the aversives position. In January 1990, the AAMR board of directors approved a revised policy statement developed by the task force. While those who supported the continued use of aversives had certainly hoped that AAMR would temper its position on these approaches in the revised statement, the Association did no such thing. The original language was largely unchanged, and AAMR retained its explicit condemnation and call for the elimination of "inhumane forms of aversive procedures."[21] Two additional paragraphs were included to clarify the values and goals that lay behind it. The task force highlighted AAMR's desire to encourage the field towards developing nonaversive alternatives, while working to enhance the empowerment and integration of people with mental retardation in community settings. After careful reconsideration, AAMR's categorical rejection of aversives remained, and the Association chose to double down on the values that informed it.

Along similar lines, in 1987 TASH published the book *Use of Aversive Procedures with Persons who Are Disabled*, coauthored by four special educators, including Turnbull. The monograph further developed and supported TASH's resolution on aversives. A review of the academic literature showed that aversives were primarily used on people with "severe" mental retardation or autism with emotional disturbances. The authors readily acknowledged that many of these studies had found aversives to be clinically effective—at least in the short term—in reducing some behaviors. However, they held that efficacy was beside the point, since aversives were painful, dehumanizing, and stigmatizing toward disabled people—and thus unacceptable. While some supporters suggested that aversives helped to facilitate community integration by reducing undesirable, destructive, or self-injurious behaviors, TASH argued that the continued use of aversives did even more to *negatively* affect professional and societal views of disabled people.[22]

Around this time, clinical psychologist James Mulick emerged as one of the most vocal defenders of applying B. F. Skinner's behaviorist theories in developing interventions for individuals with intellectual and developmental disabilities, including the continued value and use of aversives for behavior modification. Mulick had experience with the use of aversive procedures and was convinced of their transformative value in diminishing self-injurious behavior among autistic people and individuals with intellectual disabilities. He believed that these interventions could help facilitate moving people with "severe" developmental disabilities from institutions to their local communities, including enrollment in public schools.[23]

Mulick could cite his own anecdotal success stories that involved the use of aversives on people with "severe" disabilities and was impressed by other reports of major achievements. For instance, Linscheid's application of electroshock to an infant over ten days to stop ruminative vomiting, after which the child gained weight and continued "normal" development.[24] In these cases, aversive procedures were used on nonverbal individuals to bring about what appeared to be positive and long-term behavioral changes, which facilitated further functional advancements.

It is important to note that this concept of "severe" disabilities was and is more of a value judgment than an objective category. Disabled people have a wide spectrum of experiences, some of which are more difficult, potentially dangerous, or medically involved—at least for a time. Postwar clinicians and bioethicists often pointed to assessments of severity in making their recommendations. The label of "severe" could have horrendous implications for disabled people in its use to justify dismissive, painful, dehumanizing, or nihilistic responses and interventions.[25]

In 1990, Mulick published a review of TASH's monograph on aversives in which he sought to distinguish "scientific perspectives" from "ideological perspectives." He characterized science as "an approach to knowing things that has evolved a set of methods to make valid observations and test conclusions. Science, moreover, is a way of generating new knowledge, whereas ideologies are used to organize and actualize the things their adherents feel they already know."[26] With this construction of pure science as progressive and disinterested—in comparison to the reification of preconceived notions by social and political ideologies—Mulick sought to defend the dominant role of psychologists' scientific methodologies and clinical assessment.

Mulick presented "ideology" as a barrier to progress, noting that new scientific findings often challenged prevailing ideological notions. Attempting to turn the tables on TASH's arguments, he proposed, "The moral question that is of greatest importance . . . involves the price we and our clients should be willing to pay for the luxury of adhering to moral and ideological absolutes that prevent the use of some of the effective treatments that behavioral science makes available."[27] In doing so, he added to other clinical psychologists' arguments that TASH and AAMR's opposition to aversives would deprive people of a "right to effective treatment."[28]

Several responses to Mulick critiqued his framing of the aversives debate as a clash between science and ideology. Special educators Norris G. Haring (a cofounder of TASH) and Owen White suggested that both sides made ideological arguments. While TASH's monograph held that aversives were unacceptably inhumane even if they were effective, Mulick embraced an ideological position privileging "the achievement of the fullest human potential"—using aversives, if necessary. Haring and White argued that "advocates of the TASH position appear to have made a tactical error by referring to research; and persons opposed to the TASH position have made the inferential error of assuming that such a reference means that research could change the TASH position. It cannot. Only ideological arguments can ever change fundamental ideological stances."[29] This was a battle of ideologies, not of science versus nonscience.

Mulick had broader professional concerns related to the aversives controversy. Along with his frequent intellectual collaborator, research psychologist John W. Jacobson, Mulick wrote a regular column in the APA Division 33 newsletter. Here they described, with great concern, the growing involvement of disability professionals in what they called "social advocacy, in which the instrumental purpose of the advocacy behavior is to assert the rights of a group of people, rather than a specific individual." Mulick and Jacobson distinguished "social advocacy" from self-advocacy and family advocacy, noting that the former addressed "abstract entities, rather than real people."[30] As they saw it, social advocacy was an inappropriate and potentially harmful role for clinical psychologists and developmental disability specialists. They presented social advocacy as a largely verbal and highly social and uncritical activity, which made professionals feel good in pursuing idealistic goals to change the wider world but which also critically diminished their scientific role and identity.

Mulick and Jacobson's views on "social advocacy" paralleled the hesitations and concerns—that I address in this book—of other clinical professionals who tended to view their appropriate professional advocacy role as narrowly limited to clinical settings and working with specific individuals and families (chapters 1 and 3). As I describe, many clinical practitioners saw advocacy efforts that encouraged more positive, inclusive, and sociopolitical views of disabled people as inappropriate, misleading, or biased. Along these lines, Mulick and Jacobson characterized "social advocates" as working to change society—with or without empirical evidence to support their ambitions. As they put it, "Social advocacy encourages the public adoption of a perspective of optimism (e.g., empowerment, rights assertion), rather than skepticism (e.g., scientific proof)."[31] Their critique was similar to clinical psychologist Edward Zigler's 1976 denunciation of normalization as being "a banner in search of some data."[32] In these cases, psychologists lamented the incursion of "social advocates" into their expert domain and presented these advocates' ambitions as dangerously lacking a sober awareness of real-world challenges and limitations for people with intellectual and developmental disabilities.

Especially in the context of aversives, the sense of embattlement that psychologists felt was summed up by Jacobson, who cautioned, "Psychologists can be essentially eliminated from participation in the debate if advocates offer only those arguments that are not subject to appraisal within a scientific paradigm, or if they are successful in disenfranchising the scientific paradigm as a relevant model."[33] Psychologists had no ground to stand on if their scientific expertise and identity was diminished in relevance and prestige. Thus, protecting the power and legitimacy of scientific methodologies in the developmental disabilities area was critical to maintaining psychologists' seat at the table. AAMR's policy shift on aversives was an ominous sign. The Association was a long-standing professional home—along with APA Division 33—for clinical psychologists who studied intellectual disabilities, but AAMR's leaders were shifting away from prioritizing scientific investments and considerations.[34] As president, Turnbull had an advocacy-focused view of AAMR's primary identity, stating, "I advocate because all professional activity is but a means, not an end. Science for its own sake does not justify science."[35]

Clinical psychologists saw many reasons to be worried about maintaining the privileged status of their theories and techniques within AAMR and the broader developmental disabilities area. Many APA Division 33 members believed that their primary recourse—beyond abandoning the Association altogether—was to make a concerted stand for the continued priority of scientific understandings and approaches in developmental disabilities, against the growing influence of "social advocacy." As I describe in the next sections, the concerns of some psychologists about their future place and influence within AAMR continued to compound during the 1990s, with the development of a newly revised manual on classification and terminology in mental retardation.

A New Approach to Classification

In the May 1993 issue of APA's professional newsletter, the *Monitor*, a quote from John Jacobson used unusually derisive language to describe the new edition of a prominent and long-standing reference book in the mental retardation field. He stated, "The new AAMR manual is a political manifesto, not a clinical document."[36] Jacobson was leading the attack on the recently published ninth edition of AAMR's *Mental Retardation: Definitions, Classification, and Systems of Supports* (hereafter, the 1992 manual). In print since 1921, AAMR's manual on terminology and classification was, and still is, widely recognized as the definitive professional guide to understanding and diagnosing intellectual disabilities in the United States and internationally.

Vigorous disputes over the classification of mental retardation in the 1990s reveal some of the challenges involved in encouraging the adoption of new, more positive, inclusive, and sociopolitical views of developmental disabilities among clinicians and scientists. Clinical psychologist critics of the 1992 manual held that professional practice and new directions in the intellectual and developmental disabilities area should be both driven and structured by empirical research and subjected to quantitative scientific validation. Many of the 1992 manual authors were themselves outward supporters of such scientific methods. However, they also strongly believed that other values, methods, and goals could play a leading role in the development of new understandings and approaches to intellectual disabilities. I explore the evolving tensions and negotiations concerning the degree to which scientific measures and methods could be productively aligned with more positive and inclusive perspectives in disability classification.

The 1992 manual revision committee was primed for reform from the beginning. In the late 1980s, Turnbull was integral to shaping the group's orientation. He tapped lawyer and special education professor Ruth Luckasson to chair the committee and to choose its members. Luckasson had extensive personal experience with intellectual and developmental disabilities. She grew up on the grounds of a residential institution in New Mexico during the 1950s and '60s, where her father ran a dairy barn. From a young age, she engaged with many of the residents and became a long-standing advocate on their behalf as a disability rights lawyer.[37]

Luckasson chose three psychologists for the committee, including Jack Stark, a clinician whose son had significant intellectual and developmental disabilities following a nearly fatal meningitis infection. In the 1970s, Stark had worked closely with psychiatrist Frank Menolascino and clinical psychologist Wolf Wolfensberger, who together had led Nebraska's revolutionary transformation away from institutions to community services (chapter 1).[38] Stark and one other revision committee participant, clinical psychologist Steven Reiss, were also members of APA Division 33, which eventually aligned against their work.[39] Luckasson also recruited Nebraska-based psychologist Robert Schalock, as well as David Coulter, a child neurologist. Coulter credited his wife, Mary Cerreto—herself a clinical psychologist and vocal proponent of normalization and complete deinstitutionalization during this period (chapter 1)—for sparking his interest in developmental disabilities, an area that child neurologists often avoided (chapter 5).[40]

Over four years, the revision committee met frequently to formulate the 1992 manual. Schalock later noted, "It was just one of those times that were right to rethink the whole field. . . . We saw the potential of shifting the paradigm to a developmental model and a supports-based service delivery system. . . . [The 1992 Manual] really was a major revolutionary step in how people conceived of intellectual disability."[41] Based in part on their personal knowledge and engagement with children and families with developmental disabilities, the committee members sought to reorient conceptions of mental retardation away from being viewed as an individual deficit and toward being understood as the outcome of interactions between one's intellectual capabilities and social contexts. As the 1992 manual put it, "Mental retardation is not something you have, like blue eyes or a bad heart. Nor is it something you are, like being short or thin. It is not a medical disorder. . . . [It] describes the 'fit' between the capabilities of the individual and the structure and expectations of the individual's personal and social environment."[42]

In previous editions of the AAMR manual, including the most recent one in 1983, subcategories of mental retardation—mild, moderate, severe, and profound—were determined by a single quantitative measure: IQ score. The diagnostic process also included assessment of adaptive behaviors, like communication, self-care, learning, and social skills. The 1992 manual authors chose to introduce a new system that instead classified mental retardation by the level of supports that an individual required to achieve the greatest possible degree of independence and community inclusion. The authors categorized these support levels as: intermittent, limited, extensive, and pervasive (ILEP). In downplaying the importance of IQ, they sought to increase the significance of adaptive behaviors in the new system. Ten adaptive skill areas were identified for assessment, each of which could be assigned an ILEP intensity score for support needs.[43]

While there was some overlap between the ten skills areas identified in the 1992 manual and the adaptive skill categories that had been used in earlier editions, many of the newly added areas had not previously been identified or examined by clinical psychologists—meaning that there was no quantitative data or methods available for assessing them as there was for IQ. Additionally, there was no existing scientific evidence that supported the appropriateness of distinguishing and assessing these specific ten skill areas. This lack of an empirical basis for the new classification system became a major point of contention for some clinical psychologists.[44]

Soon after the 1992 manual was published, many Division 33 psychologists challenged the basis and justification for the considerable changes that Luckasson and her committee had introduced. Jacobson argued that the revisions were "politically motivated and not based on psychology's concerns and research." Along similar lines, Division 33 President-Elect Robert Sprague noted, "No marked new treatment [has occurred] that would necessitate this radical change. It's quite a departure that is ideologically driven rather than empirically driven."[45] Many of these psychologists' objections to the 1992 manual were similar to their criticism of AAMR's revised position on aversives six years earlier. In both instances, they lamented the ideology that informed the changes and the presumed professional implications for clinical psychologists.

Jacobson and Mulick criticized the process by which the 1992 manual was developed and peer reviewed—accusing the revision committee of placing "political correctness" ahead of scientifically informed decision-making. In 1993, they wrote, "The new political correctness affirms equality in all aspects of human endeavor. . . . [This] has dramatically affected the 1992 [manual]. . . . All submissions of comments upon proposals distributed to the field were treated as equal, regardless of their source. . . . Consensus of opinion, not expertise, was the basis for responding to criticisms."[46] As Jacobson and Mulick saw it, the revision committee relegated psychologists' scientific expertise and their established approaches for measuring individual intelligence to a greatly diminished status—as just one of many relevant interest groups.

Concerned clinical psychologists argued that the 1992 manual threatened to remove the assessment of intellectual disabilities from their exclusive jurisdiction, by making it an interdisciplinary process. Matson noted, "The interdisciplinary team approach suggested by the manual . . . may be 'disastrous' for psychologists. Having to arrive at a consensus with other team members who do not have similar training or expertise will 'dramatically diminish' a psychologist's role."[47] Many of the ten adaptive skills that had been identified as relevant to diagnosis were very difficult to assess in the clinic—especially in comparison to measuring IQ. This meant that clinical psychologists would be more dependent on other professionals for input.

The 1992 manual's vociferous critics did not speak for all clinical psychologists. After all, the AAMR revision committee had three psychologists as members—who now found themselves on the frontlines of defending its new directions. Schalock recalled,

> I was the sacred cow at one of the [psychology] meetings around 1990 where we were planning to suggest that individuals should be subclassified based on support needs and not IQ levels. . . . It was not well received. . . . The pushback came from psychologists who were really concerned about what would happen to their God—IQ—if we moved toward a supports paradigm.[48]

Stark attempted to downplay the significance of the revision committee's changes, by suggesting that the actual definition of mental retardation was little changed from 1983. This was somewhat accurate, since the 1992 alterations to the definition mostly involved adding more detail about adaptive skill areas. However, Stark's claim proved difficult to maintain given AAMR's advertising campaign. In big, bold letters, ads proclaimed, "This Book Will Change the Way You Think about People with Mental Retardation," and also stated, "The old classification system is gone. The new definition classifies needed supports instead of an IQ-derived level of retardation."[49]

Indeed, the 1992 manual's contents were quite different from the previous edition. The authors highlighted four new assumptions: (1) assessment should consider cultural and linguistic diversity; (2) limits to adaptive skills take place within community-based environments; (3) deficits in some skills coexisted with strengths in others; and (4) with appropriate supports, individual functioning is likely to improve.[50] These assumptions reflected the revolutionary nature of the 1992 manual in establishing mental retardation as a status that was shaped by fluid social and environmental contexts, instead of being primarily about fixed individual deficits.

Revisions to the 1992 manual had real effects on perceptions and approaches to supporting people with intellectual disabilities. As Luckasson noted, "Parents and families were really pleased about the tone. . . . It was a positive, optimistic view of the life trajectory of people with intellectual disabilities, that with supports they could function better. . . . There was a lot of positive feedback from families, who don't usually pay that much attention to classification manuals."[51] The authors were clearly satisfied that the 1992 AAMR manual was, for the first time, more than a clinical resource for a professional audience. As they had intended, it also spoke to some of the interests and concerns of people and families with intellectual disabilities.

The 1992 manual was, on many levels, a successful revolution. It was widely accepted and adopted by clinicians, service systems, and governments. Nonetheless, the system faced significant opposition from many psychologists who opposed its new approaches because they complicated or upended existing quantitative measures. As clinical psychologist Marc Tassé, a Division 33 member and future AAMR president put it, "Introducing the concept of support needs, that was a big paradigm shift. Fast-forward 25 years and it makes a lot of sense. But back then psychologists were upset because we didn't have measures of support needs. . . . Intermittent, limited, extensive, pervasive support need levels? I don't have tools to measure that."[52] The 1992 manual was forward thinking and influential in its time, but it was also just one step in the process of reforming social and psychological conceptions of intellectual disabilities.

Calls to revise or replace the 1992 manual arose quickly, prompting even the authors to admit that they had gotten ahead of the existing science in framing the new classification system.[53] As Schalock later acknowledged, "The philosophy was there, and the commitment was there, but the science was not quite there yet."[54] Along similar lines, Coulter noted, "I have often said that the 1992 manual was poetry, the 2002 manual was the truth, and the 2010 manual was the future. . . . [The 1992 manual] was a vision. In 2002, we tried to explicate that more clearly."[55] The authors recognized that their work was far from finished and that they would need to collaborate with psychologists to empirically support and stabilize their reforms.

Meanwhile, Jacobson and Mulick responded with an effort to displace the 1992 manual altogether by successfully convincing APA to develop its own a competing text. *The Manual of Diagnosis and Professional Practice in Mental Retardation* (1996), which they edited, was strongly committed to quantitative and evidence-based approaches for diagnosis and assessment. IQ played a central role in classifying mental retardation, and the editors used precise statistical language for their assessments, stating, "For adaptive behavior measures, the criterion of significance is a summary index score that is two or more standard deviations below the mean for the appropriate norming sample."[56] The APA manual sold well but was never revised and eventually went out of print. Still, it remained an important symbol for some clinical psychologists as they worked to reassert the preeminence of their quantitative measures of individual deficits and to counter the "philosophical propensities" of the 1992 AAMR manual.[57]

Even as the AAMR manual remained the preeminent professional source for diagnosing and classifying mental retardation in the late 1990s, the authors actively engaged in revising its assumptions and approaches in ways that would satisfy a larger population of psychologists. Tassé, who had initially been a critic, went on to play a central role in revising subsequent editions. He noted, "I give the senior authors on the 1992 and the 2002 [credit], they sort of brought the wolves into the hen house to basically work together and make it better."[58]

The authors of the tenth edition, published in 2002, devoted a number of pages to listing and addressing many of the critiques and shortcomings of the 1992 manual. Among the changes for 2002 was the introduction of three new, quantitatively measurable categories of adaptive behavior: conceptual skills, practical skills, and social skills. According to Tassé, "[The ten domains] are no more. Those psychologists were right. The ten domains were not empirical. . . . [W]hen you used statistic procedures, like factor analysis, they crumbled. . . . [T]hey are not themselves robust areas."[59] As the nature of these changes attested, the 2002 manual had more of the empirical and measurable basis that clinical psychologists found lacking in the 1992 version.

Even so, the philosophical underpinnings and ambitions of the 1992 manual were largely retained in 2002. This included the classification system's emphasis on the social, cultural, and environmental contexts behind the definition of mental retardation and its focus on measuring needs and providing supports to improve individual functioning. While the levels of support intensity—intermittent, limited, extensive, and pervasive—were also retained, the authors reintroduced the option of using other approaches, such as IQ score or medical etiology, for the purpose of classification. In the end, although the 1992 manual authors who contributed to the 2002 revision readily accepted various adjustments to ease the scientific concerns of many clinical psychologists, they did not compromise on their underlying social goals for the manual.

Tracing the revision history of the 1992 manual reveals some of the fundamental challenges involved in efforts to shift scientific and clinical understandings of intellectual disabilities—to incorporate more positive, inclusive, and sociopolitical perspectives. Since many psychologists who worked in the area perceived their professional role, identity, and prestige as being bound up in the quantitative assessment of individual traits in a clinical setting, we should not be surprised that they resisted the 1992 manual authors' decision to create many new, environmentally based adaptive skill categories. Some psychologists, and especially those in APA Division 33, responded derisively, by labeling these changes from previous editions as "political" or "ideological." Their critiques were mostly accurate. The 1992 manual authors had clear and outwardly spoken sociopolitical goals for their work. Meanwhile, the psychologist critics of the 1992 manual had their own parallel ideological and political interests—rooted primarily in maintaining the status quo and with it the professional jurisdiction and established expertise that they held in the previous system, which had privileged the measurement of IQ.

Based on this historical account, we might ask: Do more inclusive and context-dependent views of developmental disabilities necessitate changes in what it means to be a psychologist or threaten the role, identity, and prestige of certain practitioners? In the case of the 1992 manual and later revisions, the answer to this appears to be no. The diverse perspectives of clinical psychologists and the willingness of some to collaborate in revision— despite their existing concerns—helped establish new approaches to understanding and assessing mental retardation, which eventually were widely— though not universally—accepted. The sociopolitical ambitions of the 1992 manual were ahead of the existing science, but the science was made to catch up.

Nonetheless, it would be naïve to presume that this is the normal way of things when sociopolitical advocacy comes into conflict with demands for empirically driven policies and evaluation. In the last part of this chapter, I examine a simultaneous controversy over autism, intellectual disabilities, and psychology. The debate over facilitated communication involved many of the same professionals, organizations, and arguments, but it played out quite differently.

Facilitating Communication?

In January 1992, AAMR promoted a talk at its upcoming annual convention by Syracuse University special educator Douglas Biklen on facilitated communication (FC), referring to the technique as "an extraordinary method, which has been very effective in aiding people with autism to communicate."[60] Biklen and many other disability advocates believed that FC allowed nonverbal autistic people, many of who were assumed to have intellectual disabilities, to speak by typing with the assistance of a facilitator. While excitement about FC grew in some circles throughout the 1990s, criticism also mounted. Skeptical courts, psychologists, and journalists questioned whether the messages conveyed in FC actually originated in the minds of individuals with developmental disabilities. Amid the expanding controversy, Biklen, FC's most prominent American supporter, and many other advocates defended the technique as an empowering outlet and lifeline for nonverbal individuals. Just as clinical psychologists argued that disabled people had a "right to effective treatment," which mandated the availability of aversives, proponents presented FC as a necessary option for supporting individuals' "right to communicate."[61]

Special educators in Australia and the United States first practiced and popularized FC during the 1970s and '80s as a way to assist people with cerebral palsy, autism, and other developmental disabilities to communicate. A facilitator placed one or both of their hands on the hand, wrist, arm, or sleeve opening of an individual to help steady and control the motion of their arm and finger as a message was typed. Sometimes, the facilitator pulled the person's arm back after each letter was pressed to slow down their motions and lessen the effects of repetitive motor ticks or compulsive actions. Each person who was facilitated responded differently to FC. Some communicated lucidly very quickly, while others took significant time to begin producing legible words and sentences. The facilitators also provided emotional support. Ideally, over time direct physical supports by the facilitator were tapered, until a hand on the shoulder and eventually no touch at all was needed for the individual to communicate through independent typing.[62]

Australian special educator Rosemary Crossley introduced Biklen to FC during his trip to Melbourne in 1989. Biklen was initially skeptical about Crossley's work, but after a second visit to Australia he became convinced of FC's immense potential value for autistic people. Soon thereafter, he introduced FC to families in Syracuse. Biklen trained many facilitators and reported success in achieving communication for the first time with many nonverbal persons.[63] He had also imported Crossley's strongly optimistic perspectives, which called for facilitators to always assume the competence of individuals—despite their clinical diagnosis and outward behaviors. Crossley argued that it was better to overestimate a person's potential and to express confidence in their ability to communicate. As Biklen described it, "Our task is not to identify or decide who cannot learn or communicate, but to try to educate and to help make communication possible. . . . Of course, we cannot be sure it will work. But it *is* important to act as if we are sure."[64] Proponents viewed the belief in one's ability to communicate, and in the FC process itself, as central to success. The mindset of providers privileged faith, hope, and perseverance.

In his 1993 book *Communication Unbound*, Biklen presented the experiential evidence that had led him to strongly believe FC allowed nonverbal autistic people to authentically communicate. Biklen characterized his research as systematic, qualitative fieldwork and presented a series of anecdotes describing his observations and interactions with multiple people being facilitated over many months. Some of these individuals transitioned over time from FC to independent communication. Others continued to rely on a facilitator, but Biklen noted that they conveyed expressions, noises, and laughter, which suggested they knew what was being typed. While many observers rejected FC's validity, proponents chose to suspend preexisting doubts about the abilities of autistic people, many of who had also been diagnosed with intellectual disabilities, and let the experience of FC speak for itself. As Biklen put it, his research on FC was about "more than issues of validity. It also concerns the social meaning of disability, the power of prevailing paradigms, the nature of science, and the difficulties of change."[65]

Responding to the doubts of other developmental disability professionals concerning FC, in particular clinical psychologists, Biklen suggested, "Regarding the literacy and ideas revealed by people using facilitated communication, at least some of the skepticism surrounding facilitated communication surely reflects the pessimistic beliefs of observers in people labeled 'disabled' and the power of ideology and hopelessness."[66] Clinical psychologists had established expertise in assessing intellectual deficits, including in nonverbal autistic people. Proponents of FC sought to change the dominant perceptions about disabled people by revealing their hidden competence and, in doing so, to convince an otherwise skeptical and pessimistic society that disabilities were not always as they appeared. These perspectives were met with significant doubt and resistance from many clinical psychologists in APA Division 33, who called for more rigorous empirical validation of FC and warned that positive testimonies based on anecdotal observations risked harming disabled people and misleading their families.

Most individuals who were undergoing FC had no formal literacy training and had never demonstrated an ability to read. So for clinical psychologists, it was incomprehensible that these people could suddenly demonstrate proficient language and literacy skills—and in some cases compose poetry. Psychologists hypothesized that the messages being typed were actually coming from the facilitators, perhaps without them even realizing it. In doing so, they pointed to previous deceits that cunning psychologists had ferreted out, including clever Hans, a horse that appeared to communicate and do simple arithmetic but in fact was responding to nonverbal cues. Suspecting a similar ruse, psychologists called for controlled scientific studies of FC.[67]

Meanwhile, proponents argued that FC revealed literacy that had been hidden by some individuals' inability to speak and their limited motor control for typing. In doing so, they drew a parallel to deaf people, who historically were misdiagnosed as having cognitive impairments because they could not hear or communicate with clinicians. Perhaps many nonverbal autistic people were also inappropriately labeled as having intellectual disabilities, when in fact they had picked up language skills from their environment, which only became apparent with FC.[68]

As FC spread from Australia to the United States in the early 1990s, the severe critiques of clinical psychologists followed. Australian psychologists Robert Cummins and Margot Prior compared FC to a parlor trick, noting that studies in Australia had generated no convincing evidence of its validity. As they put it, "'On not one single occasion' have systematic tests shown that the claimed communication actually comes from the person with the disability." Interviews with facilitators raised further doubts. One facilitator suggested that FC involved telepathy and another acknowledged that it was easier for individuals to type the correct answer when the facilitator already knew it. Clinical psychologists in the US pointed to these comments as evidence that facilitators recognized their role in generating or influencing what was typed.[69]

Jacobson, after learning in 1992 that New York State was spending millions of dollars a year on Cannon communicators—the keyboards used in FC—conducted his own scientific evaluations. He concluded that individuals only successfully answered questions when their facilitator also knew the correct response.[70] In cases where the facilitator and individual were fed different words via headphones, what the facilitator had heard was almost always typed.[71] Critics pointed to Jacobson's controlled and blinded studies as strong evidence that the messages were coming from the facilitator. FC proponents countered that people being facilitated simply did not perform well under artificial, stressful, and adversarial experimental conditions, in which fast and clear answers were expected and where surprise or deception were part of the design.[72]

In their commentaries, Jacobson and Mulick presented FC in the context of other concerning social and intellectual trends, arguing, "FC serves as a case study in how the public and, alarmingly, some professionals, fail to recognize the role of science in distinguishing truth from falsity."[73]From their perspective, FC was just another one of the many dubious "fad" interventions that existed in the developmental disabilities field.[74] Like pediatricians in previous decades (chapter 2), they noted that desperate parents and their disabled children were often victimized by these purported miracle interventions. As Jacobson and Mulick defined them, fad interventions had "an unexpected but apparently dramatic treatment response, a superficially plausible 'theory' for this effect, and a disavowal by the proponent of conventional standards of scientific procedure and proof."[75] By these standards, FC was "the ultimate fad treatment."[76]

Responding to Biklen's claim that human capabilities and experiences were not always reducible to the experimental methodologies of the natural sciences, Jacobson, Mulick, and Schwartz retorted, "Within this perspective proponents imply that all possible interpretations of human behavior have equal validity, and therefore disconfirming scientific evidence is not pertinent."[77] As with the 1992 AAMR manual, Jacobson and Mulick rejected the treatment of psychological science as just one of many competing knowledge claims in the FC debate. Explicitly linking the two simultaneous controversies, they argued, "Facilitated communication is just as much a postmodern phenomenon as the new definition of MR [mental retardation]. At the cornerstone of FC are a series of assumptions that together forms a *new way of thinking*" (emphasis in original).[78] They viewed the rise of postmodern thinking in academia, more generally, as undermining the status of controlled scientific studies.

Wayne Sailor, a cofounder of TASH, was a lone voice among clinical psychologists in supporting more open-minded approaches to assessing FC. In 1996, he argued, "A postmodern position would call for a reexamination of the premise of communication and the selection of epistemology would be governed by pragmatic concerns. Under these terms, positivistic methods can be deemed as legitimate as any others within the modern epistemologies." Sailor defended the practical value of taking multiple ways of knowing into consideration, including subjective studies. He suggested that FC might be effective for autistic people "under some conditions, at least some of the time."[79] Reflecting on the polarization over FC, he later noted, "[FC] became too much of a political issue, it was more emotional than scientific. It was the positivists blasting the [qualitative] constructivists." As Sailor saw it, if and when FC was offered, "it needs to be provided quietly, carefully, but rigorously monitored, because it is easily compromised." To openly promote FC, he stated, "will destroy you professionally."[80] Any association with FC left one open to attack—due to strong scientific opposition, as well as concerns about abuse.

Opponents particularly highlighted frequent accusations, alleged through FC, of sexual assault by close family members and other caregivers. In 1994, just a few years after FC was introduced in the United States, lawyer Kenneth N. Margolin documented 60 instances of sexual assault allegations originating from FC. All of these allegations were eventually dismissed by judges, but sometimes only after extended periods of uncertainty, separation, stigma, and significant financial costs for accused family members. Sexual assault targeting disabled individuals was, and is, widespread and disproportionately common, so it is not surprising that prosecutors initially took these allegations very seriously. Ultimately, though, because efforts to scientifically validate FC in controlled settings continuously failed, courts felt unable to discern legitimate accusations from those that had been generated, whether knowingly or not, by FC facilitators.[81]

The apparent frequency of sexual assault claims made with FC was used by its opponents, with significant success, to further dismiss the technique and, along with it, the potentially real accusations of disabled individuals. FC proponents were sensitive to this line of attack and sought to downplay the prevalence of allegations, by calling into question whether they were actually so common. They also suggested that adequate safeguards were already in place to prevent facilitators from generating false claims. When seemingly legitimate charges did occur, FC proponents argued that the criminal justice system was equipped to handle them.[82] Speaking to this issue in 2015, the leaders of TASH noted, "Virtually no intervention is risk-free. . . . [I]mportant questions are how to mitigate risk and how to fully inform parents and people with disabilities about potential risks."[83] Supporters of FC believed that the risk of misunderstandings or false accusations should not be used as a reason to deny already-marginalized individuals the dignity and autonomy that FC could provide, or as another strategy to delegitimize the technique.

TASH's "Resolution on the Right to Communicate" (2000) listed FC among the forms of augmentative and alternative communication that should be available for use by disabled individuals to express themselves. However in 2016, a diverse group of TASH members—including prominent supporters and former users of FC—chose to remove specific reference to FC from the Resolution. The group publicly circulated a cover letter explaining their decision and citing the long-standing controversy over FC's validity. They acknowledged that some TASH members had benefited from FC, stating, "A grounding principle of TASH is the presumption of competence and self-determination, which necessitates a willingness to consider all possibilities and provide the widest range of options of communication for all people."[84]

Special educator Robert Horner, a member of the TASH group who, decades earlier, published an open-minded commentary on FC's potential value, had recently changed course. In 2014, Horner called for TASH to withdraw its endorsement of FC, as part of demonstrating the Association's sincere commitment to the "science-based practices movement" in developmental disabilities.[85] When it came to FC, Horner's new perspective eventually won out. While TASH continued to put its values up front—supporting more optimistic, accepting views of the dignity and skills of disabled people—the lack of empirical and reproducible evidence supporting FC led TASH to remove it from an online list of endorsed augmentative and alternative communication technologies in 2016. Competing professional and advocacy concerns had always led to tensions within TASH. This time, the desire of some professionals to maintain a legitimate scientific identity for the organization carried the day when it came to no longer officially legitimating FC.

Conclusions

Debates over aversives, classification of mental retardation, and facilitated communication offer important examples of the professional and philosophical divisions that can occur when new narratives and approaches to disability are introduced and promoted within a clinical field or specialty area. In each of these cases, psychologists mounted a vigorous defense for the priority of their scientific expertise and clinical role in assessing people with intellectual and developmental disabilities, against the perceived threats of "fad" treatments, "social advocacy," and certain ideological trends. Members of APA Division 33 were particularly strong opponents of emerging alternative perspectives on disability. These psychologists were more heavily invested in behaviorist theories, quantitative measurement of intellectual capabilities, and controlled experimental methods—all of which were actively challenged by disability advocates. Amid this, many reluctant practitioners aimed to protect their scientific identity, professional jurisdiction, and the favored status of their methods within clinical and regulatory contexts.

A historical examination of how clinical psychologists broadly considered and challenged new views and approaches to intellectual and developmental disabilities reveals various sources of disagreement, as well as potential pathways to better resolving these conflicts. Division 33 psychologists often favored settling disagreements purely on the basis of scientific methods and evidence. As part of this, many viewed competing, more positive, and sociopolitical views of disability as misleading and threatening. Nonetheless, in the case of the 1992 AAMR manual, some psychologists did choose a collaborative path forward, which took many perspectives into consideration and produced an outcome that some professionals from all camps could support.

Similar collaborative engagement regarding aversives and FC might have quickly narrowed their uptake. FC could have been adopted more widely but with an established set of guidelines in place. Collaborating clinicians might have defined a specific end goal of fully independent communication and required immediate cessation if this was not quickly achieved. For aversives, clinical psychologists could have agreed to only use these interventions for a brief period to suppress particular behaviors and worked collaboratively toward transitioning the field to nonaversive alternatives. More open-minded approaches to each would have respected the experiences and optimism of supporters, as well as the concerns and skepticism of opponents.

Ultimately, ongoing professional controversies and the lack of diverse cooperation on aversives and FC likely contributed to the continued use of each into the 2000s—with limited oversight and sporadic regulation. It was not until the 2010s that the adoption of aversives in developmental disabilities largely disappeared. Mulick's last electroshock study for self-injurious behavior was published in 2004.[86] As of 2021, electroshock was used in just one, controversial facility for developmental disabilities in Massachusetts called the Judge Rotenberg Center.[87]

The breadth of the ongoing use of FC is difficult to assess, but the technique certainly continued to be adopted in the 2010s. Despite the controversies around it, some of FC's strongest proponents were appointed to prominent academic positions, including Biklen, Donald Cardinal, and Mary Falvey—who were named Dean of Education at Syracuse University, Chapman University, and California State University, Los Angeles, respectively.[88] While the absolutist opponents of FC made well-supported arguments against it, their efforts only found success among those who privileged the results of certain scientific studies—such as US courts and a growing number of professional and advocacy groups, like TASH and the American Speech-Language-Hearing Association.[89] However, anecdotal accounts of instances where FC did lead to independent communication and the chance to pursue functional and educational goals—including a college degree in a few cases—have continued to elicit hope and belief in the potential power of FC for disabled individuals, which controlled studies are unlikely to significantly diminish.[90]

Looking back, it is ironic and striking to see clinical psychologists warning so stridently about the potential harms of FC, while at the same time arguing for the necessary use of painful aversives on patients with similar conditions. The pairing of these concerns is readily explained, however, when viewed as a dual effort to defend the priority and prestige of certain scientific methods and ways of knowing. Late twentieth-century Division 33 clinical psychologists may have benefited from the insights of pediatricians, who in the 1960s were similarly concerned about desperate parents shopping around for other explanations and approaches to their child's disabilities and sometimes being lured by unproven interventions (chapter 2). Pediatricians had recommended maintaining a positive attitude about disabled children and an open mind about a young patient's potential. Perhaps if clinical psychologists in the 1990s had offered more positive and accepting narratives about intellectual and developmental disabilities, some families would have been less inclined to look for hope in the often overly optimistic promises of FC.

Privileging the practices of psychological science over the consideration of other social and political values may have had benefits for maintaining professional role, identity, and prestige, but it had limited impacts on disability-related policies and services. By the 1990s, providing support and care for people with intellectual and developmental disabilities had been transformed—through advocacy, legislation, and evolving societal views—into a fundamentally political issue. This outcome was exactly what some clinical psychologists had feared as they voiced their disapproval of new, more optimistic, inclusive, and sociopolitical narratives and approaches. By this point, whether psychologists realized it or not, the privileged position of scientific and clinical expertise in the developmental disabilities arena could no longer be presumed and exclusively relied upon to successfully push or defend a certain policy position. Indeed, similar to pediatricians in the 1970s (chapter 2), late twentieth-century clinical psychologists fell behind the political and intellectual trends of their period and were outdone by educators and other disability specialists—who successfully defined new disability narratives.

In chapter 5, I identify and examine similar themes in a case study of postwar pediatricians who specialized in developmental disabilities and child development. Once again, professional concerns about jurisdiction disrupted opportunities to pursue more positive, inclusive, and collaborative approaches to providing care and support for individuals with developmental disabilities. Importantly, as in clinical psychology, a few pediatricians willingly adopted and became prominent advocates of more optimistic, accepting, and sociopolitical views on disability, even as many of their colleagues remained reluctant to consider new perspectives.

5

Developmental Disabilities and Subspecialization in Pediatrics

In 1974, Johns Hopkins pediatrician Arnold Capute sent his draft proposal for a new subspecialty area called "developmental pediatrics" to Robert Cooke, a former colleague and mentor. Cooke had spent much of the last two decades attempting to create greater pediatrics interest in clinical service, research, and teaching on developmental disabilities (chapter 2). As part of this, he had recruited Capute to Johns Hopkins in the mid-1960s to help lead the clinical training of medical residents and fellows in the area. Capute was a strong teacher, mentor, and institution builder who had also set his sights on bringing greater prestige and opportunities to pediatricians who focused on children with developmental disabilities. Following the lead of other pediatrics fields during the 1960s and '70s, Capute believed that the establishment of a new subspecialty in developmental pediatrics would be the best path toward achieving these goals.

The medical specialty of pediatrics was established in the 1930s, as part of a social movement to care for well-children rather than focus on a specific organ system or scientific advance—like many other medical specialty boards created during that period. After World War II, most segmentation in American medicine occurred within existing specialties, by way of subboard formation. The first five subspecialties that the American Board of Pediatrics (ABP) approved were closely related to scientific fields or organ-based domains, beginning with cardiology in 1960 and including nephrology and endocrinology in the mid-1970s.[1] Adult subspecialties already existed in many of these areas, making pediatricians concerned about competition for younger patients. No adult subspecialty in developmental disabilities has ever existed, so pediatricians in this area never had serious concerns about similar competition. Nor did they benefit from having a successful subspecialty model to follow.

Through his organizational efforts, Capute sought to create a "home" for developmental disabilities specialists within an increasingly "compartmentalized" pediatrics field.[2] He believed that establishing a new subspecialty would push academic departments to hire more faculty in the developmental pediatrics area. This would create placements for his current and former postgraduate medical fellows, while also improving the training of other clinicians in developmental disabilities. Looking to make the field widely relevant to pediatric practice, Capute pitched developmental pediatrics broadly as a subspecialty in growth and development. In a 1974 draft proposal Capute argued,

> It now appears that each branch of pediatrics has been relegated to a subspecialty with the most important one—"growth and development"—left to the teachings of the pediatric generalist, psychiatrist, or members of the behavioral sciences. Since growth and development is the essence of pediatrics, it becomes mandatory that it be given the subspecialty recognition, dignity, and status that it deserves.[3]

Ultimately, Capute's broader framing for developmental pediatrics did more harm than good. By including expertise in growth and development within the purview of a subspecialty that was primarily focused on developmental disabilities, Capute inadvertently fomented a battle in pediatrics over who "owned" child development. Many general pediatricians self-identified as experts in child development and thus viewed Capute's subspecialization push as impinging on their domain. During an era in which antibiotics and vaccines were diminishing primary care pediatricians' bread-and-butter focus on acute infectious diseases, primary care pediatricians viewed developmental surveillance as an important growth area for office practice.[4]

At the same time, the academic pediatricians, behavioral scientists, and psychiatrists who already taught growth and development pushed back against Capute's claim. A decade earlier, prominent pediatrician Julius Richmond had argued that child development should be conceived of as "a basic science for pediatrics."[5] In postwar pediatrics, child development was viewed as foundational to clinical service and as a potentially prestigious new area for research. Many pediatricians considered themselves to be "developmentalists" and were very resistant to ceding this identity to a single subspeciality, especially one in developmental disabilities.[6] No other pediatrics interest groups were strongly interested in developmental disabilities, but Capute had walked into a minefield by seeking to simultaneously claim jurisdiction over child development.[7]

In this chapter, I examine Capute's quarter-century campaign to shepherd his proposed pediatrics subspecialty, later known as Neurodevelopmental Disabilities (NDD), into existence. Along the way, Capute faced resistance and competition from multiple interest groups, including another subspecialty effort in Developmental and Behavioral Pediatrics (DBP). Ultimately, the American Board of Medical Specialties (ABMS) certified both areas in 1999, after more than a decade of tensions and uncertainty. This history of contested status between two pediatrics contingents—each of which made distinctive claims to normal and atypical child development—specifically reveals why some clinicians resisted more positive and inclusive views of developmental disabilities. In this chapter, I argue that concerns related to professional identity, jurisdiction, and prestige disincentivized and distracted many pediatricians from adopting or encouraging more psychosocial, environmental, and advocacy-oriented perspectives on the understanding, care, and support of children and families with developmental disabilities.

Notably, in comparison to the other chapters in this book, disability advocacy does not figure prominently in this historical case study. To my knowledge, the internal battles that surrounded the formation of the NDD and DBP subspecialties never drew the prominent attention of parents or disability self-advocates. Indeed, disability self-advocates' more critical narratives about discrimination and oppression do not appear to have influenced NDD or DBP pediatricians during his period to the same extent that they shaped the disability-related views of some genetic counselors, medical geneticists, and clinical psychologists. Among NDD and DBP practitioners, professional considerations about expertise and identity led to polarization and hardened views, diminishing the potential for collaboration in addressing and advancing the sociopolitical interests of and community supports for children with developmental disabilities.

Still, many pediatricians during this period were involved in adopting and promoting more optimistic and inclusive disability narratives, even as these concerns were largely sidelined by pediatric subspecialty-related debates. Building on chapter 2, the final section of this chapter highlights some of the alternative pathways by which some postwar pediatricians entered disability advocacy and began to view disabled people as unique individuals to be celebrated. These pediatricians helped to encourage the important and influential narrative that patients with any form or degree of disability were more similar to, than distinct from, typically developing children.

Establishing Developmental Pediatrics

In 1965, Arnold Capute moved to Baltimore to begin an ad hoc fellowship in developmental and handicapping conditions of childhood at Johns Hopkins University. He had previously spent a decade in private practice general pediatrics, before a heart attack in his late 30s forced a career change. After his fellowship, Capute was appointed to the faculty at Johns Hopkins, as well as at the recently dedicated John F. Kennedy Institute for Habilitation of the Mentally and Physically Handicapped Child. In 1969, he became deputy medical director.[8]

"The Kennedy," as its employees often called it, was affiliated and colocated with Johns Hopkins Hospital and Medical School but remained financially distinct. Given the low status of developmental disabilities research and clinical practice in medicine generally, Johns Hopkins Pediatrician-in-Chief Robert Cooke—who played a central role in founding the Kennedy—believed that the institute would thrive only if other departments could not siphon its money.[9] Some of its funding had come from the Mental Retardation and Community Mental Health Centers Construction Act of 1963, PL 88-164 (chapter 2). The Kennedy Institute was one of the about 50 University Affiliated Clinical Facilities (UAF) for mental retardation established between 1965 and 1975.[10]

Cooke had recruited Capute to Johns Hopkins to create a postresidency, fellowship-level pediatrics training program in developmental disabilities. Pasquale Accardo, an early Kennedy Institute fellow and long-term collaborator with Capute, later noted,

> Cooke was looking for someone to work with kids with severe impairments. . . . The line was not long on anybody who is interested in this . . . especially to dedicate their career to it, and set up a training program for it. . . . In Capute, Cooke was lucky to find the perfect person to do this.

As part of his own ad hoc fellowship at Johns Hopkins, Capute spent a couple of years doing rotations through neurology, genetics, and other specialties that he considered relevant to child development. He used this training as a model for setting up the Kennedy's developmental pediatrics fellowship program.

Capute's previous education and experience was in general pediatrics. Mid-century pediatrics residency training was heavily focused on diagnosing and treating acute, infectious diseases. So, like most of his pediatrics colleagues, Capute had little to no formal training in caring for children with developmental disabilities. As Accardo put it, "Capute was in the same boat as most pediatricians, in that he didn't know squat about development."[11] Given the lack of available models for training programs in developmental disabilities at this time, Capute decided to start his own form scratch. He also chose to build the Kennedy's fellowship program around cerebral palsy (CP). Capute's early interest in CP was strongly shaped by the Kennedy's initial affiliation with the Children's Rehabilitation Institute in Baltimore, which specialized in this condition. When the Kennedy opened, the Children's Rehabilitation Institute's patients were transferred over. Capute was closely involved in their assessment and subsequent clinical care.[12]

Capute came to understand CP as the most "severe" form of a "spectrum" of developmental disabilities caused by "chronic brain damage." He viewed CP as the best model for conceptualizing the origins and continuum of impacts of neurologically based developmental disabilities generally. Capute addressed other common developmental disability diagnoses, including mental retardation, autism, communication disorders, and learning disabilities as variants or milder forms of CP.[13] In one of his letters to Cooke, he suggested that children with autism should instead "be labeled as CP—communicative perverts." Cooke was not convinced.[14]

Capute believed that when students and researchers focused on CP, they also learned about multiple related developmental disabilities. An apparent advantage of this approach, as Accardo later suggested, was that trainees left the Kennedy with knowledge and experience in multiple developmental disabilities. He noted,

> The other UAFs would focus more on mental retardation or learning disabilities. So the trainees from these programs . . . would be puzzled by kids with cerebral palsy or other developmental disabilities. Capute viewed all of these disorders as brain problems varying in severity and focus, and so the only way to train people to be comfortable with any one of these was to train them to be comfortable with all of them.[15]

Accardo and Capute's adopted approaches to developmental pediatrics generally, and CP specifically, were conspicuously theoretical. They challenged the value and accuracy of existing, "superficially rigid" diagnostic categories like mental retardation, cerebral palsy, and autism, arguing that, "significant brain damage tends to involve more than a single developmental area."[16] In textbooks they wrote together, Capute and Accardo used the metaphor of an iceberg to describe their conception of developmental disabilities. Autism or mental retardation might be the initial diagnosis suggested, but often these seemingly discrete conditions were just the tip of the iceberg, with extensive symptoms caused by chronic brain damage present beneath the surface. Capute believed that by evaluating developmental disabilities more systematically, his fellowship trainees learned to see past the "spectrum" of common but misleading diagnostic categories, to recognize a broad "continuum" of cognitive, behavioral, and motor deficits.[17]

In 1991, Capute and Accardo presented developmental pediatrics as still in its Kuhnian "preparadigmatic stage" and expressed hope that "an accurate interpretation of the organic substrate of deviance lies in the future." Continued neuroscience research on normal and "abnormal" development, they suggested, was the best path forward toward developing a "comprehensive theory" of developmental pediatrics.[18] This commitment to creating a new paradigm for neurodevelopment and related pathologies reflected Capute's strong and consistent investment in neurological perspectives on developmental disabilities. Along with this, he knew that a fully formed theoretical framework for understanding and assessing neurodevelopmental disabilities could enhance the prestige and subspeciality potential of developmental pediatrics.

Capute's desire to create a developmental pediatrics subspecialty was also influenced by his institutional context. The structure and hierarchy of the pediatrics department at Johns Hopkins was dominated by subspecialties— some of which had begun there decades earlier. It was reasonable for Capute to believe that establishing a new subspeciality could be a major vehicle for his own career advancement. Indeed, Capute understood that Johns Hopkins trained and promoted specialists not general pediatricians.[19] During his first decade in Baltimore, Capute struggled to gain sufficient status in the pediatrics department and professional recognition nationally to achieve academic promotion. Over the long term, though, Capute's strategy of focusing on subspecialty development paid off. He was eventually promoted to full professor at Johns Hopkins and was the first recipient of an endowed chair named in this honor.[20]

Seeking Recognition for Developmental Pediatrics

During the early 1970s, as Capute began his push to create a developmental pediatrics subspecialty, he attempted to collaborate with various established professional organizations. Orthopedic surgeons, who provided corrective procedures and braces, dominated the American Academy of Cerebral Palsy (AACP). Capute aimed to bring a child development perspective to CP. In doing so, he campaigned for AACP to add "Developmental Medicine" to its name. These efforts were initially pushed aside by the orthopedists, although by the end of the decade, AACP did implement the name change, as its members grew interested in developmental disabilities.[21]

Looking elsewhere, Capute presented his subspecialty idea to the American Academy of Pediatrics' (AAP) Section on Child Development and Committee on Children with Handicaps (CCWH). After meeting with Capute in 1973, CCWH created a subcommittee to draft a proposal for a new subspecialty in developmental disabilities. Cooke was an influential proponent of Capute's campaign. He wrote to CCWH, "I would hazard a guess also that in the next five to ten years, considerably greater emphasis will be placed on the field of developmental disabilities, and the professional group that exhibits leadership will be given additional opportunities to develop and expand the area."[22] As Cooke presented it, a subspecialty would demonstrate pediatricians' commitment to serving children with developmental disabilities and offer parents reassurance that their children were being cared for by properly trained physicians.

Cooke and Capute had good reason to be concerned that pediatrics lacked a solid foothold in the developmental disabilities area due to the long-standing indifference of many pediatricians toward caring for this population (chapter 2). In one of his letters to Cooke, Capute lamented the growing role of social workers and occupational therapists in the field because "there are insufficient numbers of well-trained developmentalists to coordinate and supervise the management of these children. Also, the pediatricians we are training, appear to be too sophisticated to dirty their hands with the habilitation side and they're still focusing on the diagnostic and evaluation side."[23] Many pediatricians were not interested or did not feel properly trained to provide ongoing care to disabled children after establishing a diagnosis (chapter 2).

The new subspeciality's name was another important aspect of making it palatable to most pediatricians. CCWH initially pushed for the subspeciality to be called "developmental disabilities," since "developmental pediatrics" was expected to face more pushback from other interest groups in AAP. Capute later remarked to Cooke that he preferred the more general orientation of "developmental pediatrics" and did not like the idea of being called a "developmentally disabled pediatrician."[24] He perceived that there was still a taint associated with developmental disabilities and considered various other names for the subspecialty, like "Developmentology" (because it sounded more like cardiology).[25]

Capute argued that the new subspecialty should include expertise in normal *and* atypical growth and development—to strengthen its appeal and reputation in medicine and for potential fellows.[26] Cooke cautioned that an emphasis on developmental pediatrics could be "threatening to a large part of pediatrics that thinks it is concerned with developmental problems."[27] Indeed, when AAP's Section on Child Development was consulted, there was "a hang-up on the name, many people feeling that pediatrics *is* child development and a subspecialty board would really be abnormal development" (emphasis in original).[28] Variations on this response were among Capute's most significant challenges in his push for formal certification of developmental pediatrics. Many pediatricians believed child development was a core component of their discipline not a subspecialty area.

Nonetheless, Capute was very hopeful about the potential for success.[29] In 1974, the Section on Child Development, which was the most likely contingent to derail developmental pediatrics as an incursion on their domain, expressed support.[30] Between 1973 and 1976, ABMS certified four new pediatric subspecialties—all of which were in technological, laboratory, or organ-based areas. Capute hoped that developmental pediatrics would also be among this larger wave of approvals. However, as a broad area integrating both biological *and* psychosocial orientations, the potential developmental pediatrics subspecialty faced barriers associated with being the first of its kind in pediatrics. ABP and ABMS wanted to see support expressed by multiple and diverse contingents, including behaviorists, psychiatrists, and neurologists.[31]

Capute coauthored the formal proposal for subspecialization in developmental pediatrics with Lawrence Taft, a pediatrician and neurologist at Rutgers University who became CCWH chair the next year. They argued, "This aspect of pediatrics should be given subspecialty recognition in order to promote the teaching of normal and abnormal child . . . Medical students and physicians in training must recognize that research and clinical work with developmentally disabled children is both rewarding and exciting."[32] The proposal was first circulated in 1975 and quickly generated "a tremendous reaction," with strong opposition coming from child psychiatrists.[33] Other groups pushed for the name and focus of the subspeciality to be narrowed to developmental disabilities so that it did not impinge on their subspecialty domains.

By late 1976, Taft acknowledged that objections to the developmental pediatrics subspecialty proposal within AAP and ABP were many and that the momentum behind it had waned. Despite Capute's optimism during the previous year, it did not appear that approval was on the immediate horizon—no matter what name was chosen for the subspecialty.[34] The recent flurry of pediatric subspecialty approvals in laboratory and organ-based areas was being eclipsed in the discipline by a renewed push for greater investment in primary care and psychosocial considerations, including community practice, learning difficulties, and behavior. Even with the increased pressure on pediatrics departments to focus more on primary care, developmental disabilities still appeared likely to fall through the cracks.[35] While improved primary care benefited all children, CCWH noted that many general pediatricians did not feel confident in their ability to care for disabled children. As the Committee put it, the push to improve primary care was taking place "with one exception: the handicapped child."[36]

After endocrinology was certified in 1976, additional pediatric subspecialties were not approved until the mid-1980s, and once again these were in highly technical or laboratory-based fields.[37] Capute's initial push for formal recognition officially came to an end in 1979, when ABP formally rejected his and Taft's subspecialty proposal. Echoing many of the concerns that had been brought up previously by pediatricians, ABP wrote, "The developmental physician would provide coordinated multidisciplinary, long term, comprehensive and continuous care. The description of this individual seems to fit that of a well-trained pediatrician." Capute's claim that child development was poorly taught in pediatrics, and that a subspecialty was needed to enhance coverage in this area, fell flat with those who oversaw training and certification.

ABP also argued that developmental pediatrics lacked a sufficient body of its own distinctive scientific knowledge and expertise.[38] Indeed, in comparison to the other pediatric subspecialties that were approved in the 1970s, developmental pediatrics had few traditional markers of scientific engagement—such as annual conferences and journals. By 1979, Capute had already begun to correct this shortcoming. He saw ABP's explanation as further support for a new strategy, which centered on deputizing a decade's worth of former Kennedy Institute fellows to build a more established subspecialty from the ground up. As part of this, Capute and his trainees believed that it would be necessary to double down on developmental pediatrics' neurological orientation, including staking a claim on the field's own organ—the brain. In this way, Capute's cohort of developmental pediatricians sought to establish a professional identity akin to that of cardiologists and nephrologists, as organ system–based subspecialists.

In retrospect, the failure of Capute and Taft's proposal was a significant missed opportunity, since it had the potential to establish a broad-based and relatively psychosocially and environmentally oriented pediatrics subspecialty in developmental disabilities. While the proposal faced opposition from many sides, it also had a broad coalition of supporters, including AAP's Section on Child Development and CCWH.[39] Capute had long been drawn to a strong neurological focus in his approach to developmental disabilities. However, Taft and others in CCWH and the Section on Child Development helped to enhance the potential subspecialty's psychosocial emphasis. Capute and Taft's proposal highlighted the need for developmental pediatricians to understand "the socio-cultural and environmental factors" that influenced growth and development and referred to childhood developmental disabilities as "a medico-sociological challenge."[40] With his sharp turn toward neurology after the initial proposal faltered, Capute became much less likely to look past brain damage to consider social and environmental issues.

Diverging Paths in Child Development

During the late 1970s and '80s, Capute and his acolytes transitioned from their initial proposal in developmental pediatrics toward a potential subspecialty in NDD. Capute later situated NDD's pathway to subspecialty recognition as starting during this period—erasing his previous five years of widely collaborative efforts toward a subspeciality in developmental pediatrics.[41] In doing so, he moved away from coordinating with other pediatricians who were broadly interested in child development and embraced a narrower focus on the association between chronic brain damage and developmental disabilities. At the same time, some of Capute's former subspecialty collaborators began to formulate a distinct identity and orientation and became competitors with NDD for subboard recognition—in what became a battle for jurisdiction over the area of child development and disabilities.

In 1978, Capute and his many former Kennedy Institute fellows founded the Society for Developmental Pediatrics (SDP). He later noted that "most of the efforts of the Society for Developmental Pediatrics were aimed at addressing what was perceived as the weakest link in the original proposal by encouraging further development of the research base for the field."[42] This included founding an annual research seminar, a professional newsletter, and the journal *Mental Retardation and Developmental Disabilities Research Reviews*. Capute also took his campaign on the road, to cities where he invited pediatrics department chairs out to dinner at an expensive restaurant and pitch his subspecialty. While many saw value in NDD, they often felt that their colleagues would view investment in the area negatively or believed that Capute's approach to developmental disabilities was too narrowly neurological for their program.[43]

Throughout this period, the developing field of NDD remained overwhelmingly populated by physicians who had trained with Capute at the Kennedy. When the field's first textbook, *Developmental Disabilities in Infancy and Childhood*, was published in 1991, nearly all of the 28 contributing authors were present or previous faculty members or fellows in the Johns Hopkins program. Capute even established a formal organization for his current and former trainees, the Kennedy Fellows Association, which he thought would bring its members greater recognition and prestige. Fancy dinners and an annual conference, as well as a periodical and professional society, were all part of Capute's strategy to make NDD more visible and legitimate.

Beyond proponents from the Kennedy Institute orbit, however, Capute's subspecialty vision did not appear to be spreading of its own accord. Indeed, after establishing a new Section on Children with Disabilities within AAP in 1990, the founders struggled to find pediatricians from outside of the Johns Hopkins circle to take on leadership positions.[44] That year, ABP once again turned down Capute's subspecialty proposal—this time for "neurodevelopmental disabilities in pediatrics." Notably, this time the board responded more positively to the subspecialty's legitimacy and potential. They encouraged Capute to continue building on his investments in neurology, which included his research emphasis on cerebral palsy and language disorders, as well as his efforts to attract child neurologists and the American Board of Psychiatry and Neurology (ABPN) to help develop a jointly managed NDD subspecialty.[45]

Capute characterized NDD as a variant of child neurology—a field that historically focused on acute conditions like seizures and tumors rather than on chronic neurological impairments.[46] Like most pediatricians, child neurologists had little interest in developmental disabilities, but some were beginning to perceive opportunities in the area. As Accardo, Capute, and child neurologist Michael Painter put it, "A joint approach to certification in developmental disabilities could effect a closer union and resolve the difficult issue of identifying the organ system substrate for the new subspecialty."[47] That organ was the brain, and in this regard the early 1990s was an opportune time to align with neurology. In 1989, the US Congress had declared the 1990s the "decade of the brain." Innovation and improvements in neuroimaging led to new opportunities to identify and study apparent signs of chronic, organic brain damage, which Capute viewed as fundamental to understanding the causes of developmental disabilities.[48]

Just as ABP began to acknowledge the value of a NDD subspecialty, and Capute was establishing productive relations with neurology, a new obstacle appeared on the horizon. During the previous decade, another professional interest group in pediatrics had also made moves toward staking a claim in the area of child development and had taken many similar steps as Capute in establishing distinctive research and training programs. Notably, the rise of Developmental and Behavioral Pediatrics (DBP) as a parallel subspecialty contender alongside NDD was no coincidence. DBP's leaders saw that Capute was on the doorstep of subspecialty recognition and wanted to prevent him—given his narrowly neurological focus on a limited set of developmental disabilities—from claiming broad jurisdiction over all of child development and disabilities.

DBP had its origins in the thinking and efforts of Julius Richmond and other promoters of more psychosocial and community-based approaches in pediatrics.[49] These pediatricians viewed themselves as experts in the problems of child development but tended to focus much more on environmental and behavioral challenges rather than on the neurological basis of developmental disabilities. As Accardo put it, while NDD's organ system was the brain—with a focus on chronic damage and biological problems—DBP placed an emphasis on the family and society. He stated, "We have a very organic approach, they have a very sociologic approach."[50] When it came to defining a unique professional identity for each area, NDD partisans characterized themselves as brain specialists, while DBP identified as experts in child behavior and development.

The Society for Developmental and Behavioral Pediatrics was founded in 1982, under the leadership of University of Maryland, Baltimore pediatrician Stanford B. Friedman. The organization's history and identity were immediately impacted by the similarity of its name to Capute's Society for Developmental Pediatrics, which had been incorporated four years earlier—also in Maryland. Legally, this necessitated a name change to the Society for Behavioral Pediatrics (SBP).[51] Philosophically, the need to drop "developmental" generated significant reflection and discussion. Several participants in SBP's initial meetings "felt strongly that issues of normal and abnormal development were so integral to the research and teaching activities of potential Society members, that this term should be included in the title."

On the other hand, some SBP members argued that "the term 'developmental' has come to refer specifically to the care of children who are intellectually retarded and multiply handicapped, and therefore, should not be included in the official name."[52] Many in SBP also wanted to establish their professional identity and claim jurisdiction in the broad area of child behavior *and* development. They could not overlook, though, how completely Capute had already pigeonholed the term "developmental pediatrics" as focusing primarily on children with developmental disabilities—an area that some SBP members did want to be a part of their professional identity.[53] In 1983, seeking to retain "developmental" in their organization's name and identity, SBP contacted Capute about merging the two societies, but they were rebuffed. Without their preferred name, SBP adopted the descriptive motto, "Promoting Developmental and Behavioral Research and Teaching."[54]

Along with Friedman, the founding members of SBP included pediatrician Robert Haggerty, a promoter of the psychosocially oriented field of community pediatrics; T. Berry Brazelton, a child developmental specialist and prominent public figure in pediatrics; Esther Wender, the director of behavioral pediatrics at Montefiore Medical Center in New York; and Julius

Richmond, a previous US surgeon general who had been advocating for increased pediatric investment in child development research and training since 1959.[55] DBP was always a more broad-based area than NDD ever was and, as a result, SBP had a larger and more diverse membership than Capute's SDP ever did. Behavioral pediatricians were also out ahead of SDP in achieving some of the markers associated with subspecialties. The *Journal of Developmental and Behavioral Pediatrics* became SBP's official outlet more than a decade before SDP had a similar publication, and the DBP area's first textbook, *Developmental-Behavioral Pediatrics* was published in 1983, nine years before Capute and Accardo's NDD textbook.

Still, the slightly younger SBP constantly found itself playing catch-up with Capute, especially when it came to forming a subspecialty—an ambition that was not on the radar of most SBP members in the 1980s. In comparison to the existing pediatrics subspecialties, which were associated with an organ system and were laboratory based, behavioral pediatricians prided themselves in being clinically and psychosocially oriented generalists. Rather than basic research, many academic SBP members were actively engaged in improving primary care and adolescent medicine—in part by making residency programs more outpatient and community-oriented.[56] Unlike Capute, and the subspecialities that he modeled NDD after, SBP consistently presented as a *big tent* organization, which addressed the socioenvironmental challenges and needs of children.

SBP's leaders lamented Capute's unwillingness to merge or collaborate with them, in part because his intransigence disrupted their goal of establishing a broad-based society focused on child behavior and development. In 1985, Wender stated, "Any schism between behavioral pediatrics and developmental pediatrics was most unfortunate, and every effort should be made to integrate the efforts of these two groups." Friedman similarly argued that combining developmental and behavioral pediatrics would best serve the interests of patients. He also noted that this would require "changes in fellowship training, especially an increased emphasis in psychosocial topics and skills for those trained in developmental pediatrics."[57] Indeed, SBP's leaders were more interested in *acquiring* SDP than in an evenhanded merger. Capute readily perceived this and rejected all such offers. His goal of establishing a "home" for pediatric developmental disabilities specialists would not be achieved by handing over control to SBP.[58]

Other developmental pediatricians were also resistant to SBP's overtures and skeptical of the benefits of consolidation for themselves and for children with developmental disabilities. Herbert J. Cohen, a developmental pediatrician at the Rose F. Kennedy Center UAF in New York stated, "We have a clear-cut constituency in the families of the developmentally disabled and, due to our commitment to this population, a base of funding support. Why then should we merge with the new behavioral specialists who now come to town, particularly when many of them have displayed a limited interest in children with disabilities?" Cohen, who was chair of CCWH at this time, was one of many developmental pediatricians who had trained and worked entirely outside of Capute's orbit at Johns Hopkins. He similarly questioned the newly emergent behavioral pediatricians' true interests in and commitment to children with developmental disabilities. Developmental pediatricians, Cohen suggested in 1985, were well ahead of their behavioral colleagues in establishing a distinct identity in pediatrics and in formalizing training curricula for residents and fellows in child development and developmental disabilities.[59]

In the early 1990s, as Capute's NDD proposal was moving forward, SBP leaders realized that their time to act on proposing a different subspecialty was short, before the window of opportunity closed.[60] Even as many behavioral pediatricians valued their identity at generalists, it had become an unavoidable reality in medicine that subspecialization represented a primary means of gaining academic and third-party payer recognition and support. Many SBP members were troubled by Capute's narrowly neurological approach to behavior and development and his focus on developmental disabilities. They were also concerned by the real possibility that NDD might become the only subspecialty in child development to be approved.[61] Ultimately, SBP members' desire to establish and retain some jurisdiction in the broad area of child behavior and development—coupled with a significant degree of personal and professional animosity toward Capute and his approaches—helped them to overcome their reluctance about subspecialization.

Fragmented Approaches to Disability in AAP

The growing competition between SDP and SBP spilled over into AAP during the 1990s—disrupting efforts to collaborate in the area of childhood disabilities. One point of tension was Capute's desire to have a distinct AAP section on developmental disabilities. For him, a separate section represented another clear marker of professional development toward subspecialization, as well as an established "home" for developmental disabilities specialists within the Academy.[62] SBP already had close relations with the Section on Developmental and Behavioral Pediatrics (previously the Section on Child Development). AAP also had its long-standing Committee on Children with Disabilities (CCWD, formerly CCWH). Notably, AAP committees and sections were quite distinct in their membership and function, even when they addressed a similar topic. Committee members were appointed to represent geographic regions and served limited terms, while sections had to attract members. Committees focused on policy issues and statements, whereas sections were mainly interested in professional concerns and developing educational programs for generalists and trainees.

Members of the Section on Developmental and Behavioral Pediatrics (Section on DBP) objected to Capute's request for a separate section, arguing that developmental disabilities fit within their purview. Unlike when SBP was founded, DBP specialists already controlled the domain that Capute sought and argued that his contingent should join their section. Proponents for a new section distinguished their interest in "organic problems that develop into disabilities" from the Section on DBP's focus on "behavioral issues." They argued, "While the two fields share some common ground in training and knowledge, there is a marked divergence."[63] In 1990, AAP approved a separate Section on Children with Disabilities (SCWD) on the condition that it would work closely with CCWD and broaden its focus area to include all forms of disability.[64]

AAP's decision consolidated all childhood disabilities into a single section. This was clearly an unfortunate outcome, since Capute and his contingent were quite obviously not interested in disabilities beyond a narrow spectrum of developmental conditions. Rather than incorporating more conditions, as well as behavioral and environmental considerations within NDD's primarily organic focus on developmental disabilities, the compromise further separated the broad area of childhood disabilities from the more psychosocial orientation of the Section on DBP. CCWD quickly reached out to collaborate with SCWD and encouraged the new section to take on additional topics that they considered to be important, like chronic illness in children.[65]

Despite AAP's mandate, SCWD remained focused on developmental disabilities. Addressing CCWD's request that the new section take on chronic illness, its leaders noted, "The Executive Committee is willing to incorporate this type of expertise into the leadership, but upon review of the current section membership have not been able to identify section members who fit into this category."[66] The section's chosen topic for their first AAP annual meeting educational session—which targeted general pediatricians—was cerebral palsy, Capute's main interest. In 1993, the SCWD educational program focused on communication disorders and autism—continuing a developmental disabilities orientation. With encouragement from AAP, and the looming threat that the section could be dissolved after its five-year review, SCWD chose traumatic brain injuries and hearing impairments for its next two educational sessions—topics that were not focused on developmental disabilities—leading to a 70 percent drop in attendance.[67]

Clearly, there was limited interest among general pediatricians for educational programming on any disability-related topics, and SCWD members were more likely to attend when the focus was narrowly on developmental disabilities. James Perrin, who was chair of CCWD at this time, recalled of SCWD, "The Section had for years been dominated by the very good but fairly focused group at the Johns Hopkins Kennedy Institute, which does fabulous work, but is pretty narrowly focused on neurodevelopmental disorders. Most of the leaders of the section were from Kennedy, and in the early days it never developed much diversity."[68]

Meanwhile, SCWD's relations with the Section on DBP immediately turned acrimonious. In November 1991, AAP organized a "consensus conference," bringing together representatives from each section to discuss their similarities and differences. The meeting was not productive. SCWD leaders later described it as "a thoroughly political activity that produced significant animosity and wounds that have yet to heal . . . [and] only further inflamed tensions." At least one side felt very threatened by the conversation. In the SCWD executive committee's account of the conference, the Section on DBP's name was actually written in all lowercase letters and in a noticeably smaller font—literally belittling their rival's identity. SCWD leaders also noted that, while their original section proposal had intended to create a "home" for developmental disabilities specialists, AAP had betrayed their contingent with a "watered down mixed-bag section."[69]

These expressions of anger, which appeared in SCWD meeting minutes from two years after the "consensus conference," demonstrated the intense and long-standing disregard that some in SCWD felt toward the Section on DBP. The leaders of SCWD during its early years—most of who had trained with Capute—were engaged in a campaign to forge an isolated and protected place for pediatricians interested in developmental disabilities, ultimately via subspecialization. Importantly—as SCWD remained largely focused on developmental disabilities, subspecialty recognition, and feuds with the Section on DBP—it was CCWH and the Medical Home Project Working Group that encouraged collaboration and led the way in AAP on addressing policy and community-based concerns that were broadly relevant to childhood disabilities (chapter 2).

In 1993 Capute received another rejection letter from ABP. This time, the board wrote that NDD had "swung the pendulum too far toward making . . . neurodevelopmental disabilities a straightforward subdiscipline of child neurology, and in the process lost emphasis on the psychosocial, behavioral, and chronic disease."[70] Sensing another opportunity for acquisition, SBP leaders once again reached out to suggest a merger. Capute refused, pointing as always to the significant differences in their perspectives.[71] By this time, Capute's transition away from his initial developmental pediatrics proposal in the 1970s was irreversible. He was fully committed to a resolutely neurological vision and resisted any attempts to dilute his NDD approaches within the more psychosocially oriented DBP subspecialty. Capute's persistence and immovability were highly regarded by his Johns Hopkins trainees and colleagues. All three of the ABP rejection letters Capute received, between 1979 and 1993, were framed and have been displayed for decades in the Kennedy Institute—as battle scars and monuments to his long battle for recognition.[72]

Negotiating for Two Distinct Subspecialties

A medical subspecialty is fundamentally defined by its distinct body of scientific and clinical knowledge and expertise. Capute and his former fellows spent decades establishing a scientific basis for the NDD subspecialty, highlighting neurology and organic brain damage. As the DBP subspecialty push picked up steam in the mid-1990s, some practitioners suggested that SBP similarly needed to develop and promote a more rigorous scientific identity. Jack Shonkoff, a developmental pediatrician and DBP partisan who had trained at Boston Children's Hospital, likened the situation to the "soft" sciences seeking to gain acceptance in a context dominated by the "hard" sciences. He encouraged developmental and behavioral pediatricians to embrace a more "hard-nosed science" demeanor, characterized by "constructive skepticism and critical self-evaluation," as well as to more actively assimilate developmental disabilities into DBP's domain.[73]

Historically Shonkoff noted, children with "severe" disabilities were seen as "so different from the general population (and met so inadequately) as to justify substantially separate clinical and educational services. That legacy of a separate service system is perpetuated by some thoughtful advocates dedicated to the care of children with severe disabilities, as well as by others who eschew such responsibilities." Shonkoff believed that a separate sub-specialty for children with developmental disabilities was backward looking and critiqued his SBP colleagues who were willing to leave children with developmental disabilities outside of their purview. Just as distinguishing "behavioral" from "developmental" pediatrics or "soft" and "hard" sciences was unproductive, he argued that drawing lines and dividing disabled children between two subspecialties based on their perceived level of "severity" was no longer appropriate.[74]

Despite Shonkoff's entreaties, many DBP practitioners were satisfied with claiming jurisdiction over a specific domain defined by patients at "the low-severity, high prevalence end of the developmental / behavioral spectrum," with attention deficits and hyperactivity.[75] Members of SBP expressed concern about whether this range of conditions would be covered by the new health care plans being put forth by the Clinton Administration in the early 1990s. High-severity, low prevalence conditions, like cerebral palsy and intellectual disability, were perceived as more likely to be covered, but fit more comfortably in NDD's domain. Even with their focus on "low-severity" conditions, it was common for DBP practitioners to engage in multihour patient meetings, for which they struggled to receive adequate compensation.[76] DBP proponents believed that subspecialty status would give them more influence in addressing such issues.[77]

Capute's NDD contingent was similarly active in defining and distinguishing their patients and domain of expertise—by highlighting a strong commitment to more "severe" developmental disabilities. In 1995, SCWD noted that its members were "better suited to cover more controversial issues such as autism, cerebral palsy, etc. The Section on Developmental and Behavioral Pediatrics is better suited to education on behavioral issues."[78] This characterization at once situated SCWD as taking on children with conditions that were often stigmatized and purposely relegated DBP practitioners to managing conditions that were less obviously medical.

Meanwhile, DBP proponents characterized their interests as more in line with those of general pediatricians and critiqued NDD's limited focus on children with high-severity, low prevalence neurologically handicapping conditions.[79] Notably, as Capute and colleagues moved closer to identifying with neurology and developmental disabilities, SBP reclaimed the word "developmental," becoming the Society on Developmental and Behavioral Pediatrics (SDBP) once again in 1995. As the DBP subspecialty campaign continued, SDBP retained their *big tent* identity, highlighting a biopsychosocial orientation and wide-ranging patient population. In 1997, SDBP President Peter Gorski acknowledged that this included the desire to "own" specific developmental disabilities, such as attention deficit disorder.[80] While proponents of DBP were willing to dispense with the neurodevelopmental disabilities that most interested Capute and his fellows, they were also interested in staking a claim on more prevalent behavioral conditions.

Over time, some pediatricians who specialized in developmental disabilities, but had trained outside of Capute's orbit, also gravitated to SDBP. For example, F. Curt Bennett, who did a fellowship in child development and handicaps at the University of Washington, had interests and expertise that were more closely aligned with NDD but was turned off by Capute's narrowly neurological approach to developmental disabilities. As incoming president of SDBP in 1996 he stated, "It is now more imperative than ever that we are ultimately successful in obtaining [DBP] subspecialty status and an alternative pathway within pediatrics for our inclusive and broadly envisioned field." Tina Iyama, a developmental pediatrician who trained at the University of Wisconsin, wrote in a critical review of Capute and Accardo's textbook, "We must abandon our preconceived notions of what 'belongs' and 'does not belong' to developmental pediatrics and embrace the broadest possible concept . . . that we as specialists in development can be of service to all children."[81] Similarly, developmental pediatrician Herbert Cohen, who had once supported Capute's developmental pediatrics subspecialty push, admitted, "The decision to merge NDD with pediatric neurology is probably the only major thing about which Arnold and I disagreed."[82]

Beyond pediatrics, the evolving scope of both NDD and DBP came to the attention of another medical specialty board, the American Board of Psychiatry and Neurology (ABPN). Capute's maneuvers to create NDD required significant negotiations with neurologists. One complication involved training in child neurology, which neurologists believed should include significant time working with adult patients as well—a requirement that did not appeal to many pediatricians who were specifically interested in children with developmental disabilities.[83]

Meanwhile, child psychiatrists opposed the DBP subspecialty, presenting it as an incursion into their jurisdiction of child mental health and threatening to weaken their training programs and create confusion for patients. The Section on DBP retorted that there were already "more children with a variety of emotional-behavioral-developmental-social problems than either pediatricians or psychiatrists can handle alone" and suggested that "political and financial defensiveness" were clearly behind child psychiatrists' resistance.[84] SDBP President Ellen Perrin expressed hope that ABPN would appreciate DBP's distinctiveness from child psychiatry. As she put it, "We hope to reassure them [ABPN] that we are not, in fact, attempting to compete with child psychiatrists, but to create a different sort of professional who would collaborate with child psychiatrists and with child neurologists, as well as with general pediatricians."[85]

While some child psychiatrists resisted a new subspecialty in DBP, many general pediatricians were onboard. Surveys of academic and community pediatricians during the mid-1990s found that most did not feel threatened by DBP and valued the improved training and research that the subspecialty would facilitate.[86] This was a notable change from the 1970s, when many general pediatricians viewed a subspecialty in developmental pediatrics as an incursion on their domain. General pediatricians may have also felt more comfortable with the broad scope and patient population of DBP, relative to the narrow focus on developmental disabilities that Capute had initially envisioned for developmental pediatrics. By the 1990s, demand vastly outstripped supply when it came to caring for children with developmental and behavioral conditions. General pediatricians were thus happy to collaborate with specialists in this area.

In 1996, ABP indicated its support for Capute's NDD proposal, as long as the new subspeciality was primarily administered by ABPN. This would open the door for ABP to oversee the DBP subspeciality. The overarching American Board of Medical Specialties (ABMS) ultimately approved this arrangement in 1999, creating two new subspecialties. The certification of NDD was a significant victory for Capute and his ever-growing cohort of Kennedy Fellows, following a quarter century of challenges, competition, and frequent rejection. Years of struggle had produced a complex end result, which was neurologically focused—as Capute had long envisioned—but also outside of the immediate oversight of pediatrics, where he had begun. The NDD training process involved two years of pediatrics residency, followed by one year of adult neurology, 18 months of child neurology and developmental pediatrics, and 18 months of neurosciences and research. NDD fellows were then eligible to be "triple boarded" in pediatrics, neurology, and NDD.[87] DBP had a more traditional training model, with three years of pediatrics residency and three years of DBP fellowship.

During their first two decades, both subspecialties were significantly understaffed.[88] NDD's unusual "2-4" approach (two years of residency and four years of fellowship) created a notable barrier to entry, by requiring the transition from pediatrics residency to a neurology fellowship after just two years instead of the normal three. This meant that potential trainees had to commit and apply to NDD very early in their residency experience. These complexities, coupled with the NDD subspecialization requirement of one year of training in adult neurology, contributed to disappointing recruitment over the years. DBP also experienced suboptimal recruitment. For some potential fellows, the three-year commitment to additional training after residency did not promise a sufficient return on investment, especially in a subspecialty that involved long patient visits and relatively poor compensation. The third year of DBP fellowships were required to have a research focus. For pediatricians who were more interested in the clinical aspects of DBP, this was a disincentive.[89]

Would the picture have looked different if NDD and DBP had consolidated into one subspecialty? The answer to this question is anyone's guess. When it came to pediatricians who were specifically interested in developmental disabilities, the two subspecialties were likely competing with one another for the same fellows. Indeed, potential trainees often experienced some degree of confusion about which pathway to follow.[90] A number of pediatricians who specialized in developmental disabilities, and especially those who trained before 2000, ended up getting certified in both areas once they were created. Some even moved between NDD and DBP positions during their careers—showing the real-world overlap and fluidity between the two subspecialties.

At the organizational level, AAP's CCWD and SCWD combined to form the Council on Children with Disabilities in 2005, under the leadership of pediatrician Paul Lipkin—a Capute trainee and partisan who was board certified in both NDD and DBP. While SDP folded after its primary goal of a NDD subspeciality was achieved, SDBP continued to exist, as did the separate AAP Section on DBP—which Lipkin eventually joined (after someone offered to pay his dues). These groups worked together on many projects during the 2000s, including an effort to improve developmental screening criteria. Amid this, Lipkin admitted to remaining somewhat territorial and partisan. As chair of AAP's collaborative developmental screening project, he successfully resisted the inclusion of the word "behavioral" in the final product's title.[91] Indeed, long-standing professional allegiances and identities lingered, even as outward polarization began to recede.

Conclusions

Sociologist Andrew Abbott has argued, "A profession is not prevented from founding a national association because another has one. It can create schools, journals, ethics codes at will. But it cannot occupy a jurisdiction without either finding it vacant or fighting for it."[92] When Arnold Capute first sought to establish a new subspeciality in the 1970s, the area of pediatric developmental disabilities was vacant, and yet he still ended up fighting for this domain due to his insistence on also incorporating the broader area of child development. After the initial rejection of developmental pediatrics, Capute and his Johns Hopkins fellows worked to establish many of the traditional markers of subspecialty status, including societies, textbooks, and conferences. Through these efforts, they raised the recognition and prestige of research and service in pediatric developmental disabilities and established a lasting theoretical framework for the area.[93] However, Capute never managed to gain ground in the larger jurisdictional battle that he had helped to instigate over who "owned" child development within pediatrics. Ultimately, the Johns Hopkins contingent had to move outside of the formal boundaries of the pediatrics specialty to achieve a lasting claim over the domain of child development, within neurology.

In retrospect, the rejection of Capute's initial developmental pediatrics subspecialty proposal was a major missed opportunity for establishing broad-based training programs and professional expertise among specialists in developmental disabilities. Despite his long-standing preference for neurological perspectives, during the mid-1970s Capute had demonstrated openness to making developmental pediatrics more psychosocially oriented. Indeed, the original developmental pediatrics proposal was built on significant consensus—drawing support from the AAP Committee on Children with Handicaps and the Section on Child Development. Its failure amid jurisdictional competition over child development hardened Capute's resolve to follow an organ-based approach to establishing NDD's professional identity and achieving greater prestige as a recognized subspecialty. Capute's neurological turn, coupled with many DBP proponents' tepid interest in children with developmental disabilities—and their desire to maintain a broader identity as experts in behavior *and* development—impeded any chances for future collaboration.

Throughout this book, I examine the various professional reasons why clinicians adopted, promoted, or resisted more optimistic and accepting narratives of disability. Notably, Capute and many other NDD subspecialty proponents did not actively respond to or reject more positive and inclusive views of developmental disabilities because, for the most part, these concepts were not even on their radar. Rather, many of NDD's basic tenets directly countered more optimistic and sociopolitical perspectives on developmental disabilities. For instance, Capute characterized patients with developmental disabilities as "brain damaged persons" and focused on improving the biomedical understanding, assessment, diagnosis, and amelioration of their "pathological" conditions. One of Capute's best-known aphorisms among his fellows, whether they agreed with it or not was, "You can't make a race horse out of a pig."[94] With it, he pessimistically foregrounded perceived biological limitations and privileged medical expertise over considering socioenvironmental factors. This aphorism also clearly revealed his personal attitudes about certain disabled people. Importantly, though, these views cannot be neatly disentangled from his professional interests in seeing disability as a fixed, individual deficit.

Capute was not a societal and political reformer, but he was an institution builder. One of his major goals was to improve the professional circumstances and opportunities for NDD fellows, so that they could provide better care for children with developmental disabilities. In Capute's view, the fact that NDD pediatricians were *at all* interested and willing to commit to doing research and providing care related to developmental disabilities was a major step forward for disabled children and their families—relative to the broader field of pediatrics.

As part of this, many NDD adherents dismissed DBP practitioners as not truly invested in children with developmental disabilities. Their concerns were, to a certain degree, well founded. DBP was always more of a *big tent* organization, and the potential for developmental disabilities to receive less attention within the subspecialty area was real. While some DBP partisans did specialize in developmental disabilities, most did not, and a few even resisted the inclusion of developmental disabilities into the DBP domain. When DBP wrote its first certification exam in the early 2000s, "cognitive / adaptive disabilities" and "motor disabilities and multiple handicaps" were included but comprised less than 10 percent of the total contents.[95] In comparison to NDD training, DBP programs valuably included more socio-environmental perspectives on child behavior, development, and disability. However, DBP practitioners did not always view these approaches as equally applying to children with more "severe" developmental disabilities.

Children and families with developmental disabilities may have benefited from greater collaboration between NDD and DBP, especially if it had led to more diverse perspectives—beyond a narrowly neurological orientation—on developmental disabilities. From a professional viewpoint, however, Capute's continual rejection of a merger between NDD and DBP proved—in the end—to be strategically savvy and successful. Capute's persistence certainly benefitted his career and brought wider and better-established recognition and status to NDD subspecialists.[96] At the same time, it is clear that the push among some DBP partisans to merge with NDD was not primarily about keeping developmental disabilities within DBP or preventing this area from being shifted over to neurology. Rather, integration was a means to regain and stabilize DBP's jurisdictional claim on child development, while easing the pathway to subspecialty recognition.

It is unfortunate, yet unsurprising, that professional considerations and stakes were so central to the positioning of, and investment in, developmental disabilities in late twentieth-century pediatrics. A single subspecialty that addressed developmental disabilities from a diversity of perspectives—biological, psychosocial, environmental, and political—likely would have been better for promoting more positive and inclusive disability narratives. There is no way to know if such an outcome would have been possible in the absence of Capute's obduracy and other pediatricians' desire to protect their jurisdiction over other approaches to child development. Luckily, as I describe below, internecine professional battles over subspecialization did not completely overshadow some pediatricians' advocacy efforts in developmental disabilities.

Coda: Alternative Approaches to Disability in Pediatrics

Compared to behavioral and neurodevelopmental disabilities specialists, postwar pediatricians who specialized in genetically discrete conditions primarily steered clear of the subspecialty quarrels over child development and disabilities. Interestingly, the pediatric medical geneticists that I interviewed for this project expressed some of the most sociopolitically oriented and progressive perspectives on disabilities issues, compared to other pediatricians. For me, this was initially a surprising finding, given the specific focus of medical geneticists on very specific, biological causes of certain disabilities. I attribute this anecdotal finding to a variety of factors.

Postwar medical geneticists had close working relationships with disabled children and their families, including partnerships in developing and leading advocacy groups like the 22q11.2 Syndrome Foundation, National Down Syndrome Society, and SOFT (chapters 3 and 6).[97] Some medical geneticists also began their careers working in hospitals and residential institutions, where they experienced firsthand the dehumanization of children with supposedly "severe" or "hopeless" disabilities.[98] In addition to this, as I describe in chapter 6, many medical geneticists were directly targeted by disability self-advocates, who sought to introduce new narratives of disability into medicine and who were particularly troubled by the proliferation of prenatal testing and selective abortion. These advocates strongly influenced some medical geneticists, leading them to adopt more positive and inclusive views of disability, alongside biomedical conceptions.

It is important to note that medical geneticists were not weighed down in the same way by professional concerns over identity, jurisdiction, and medical subspecialty recognition as were their NDD and DBP colleagues. Indeed, they faced little clinical competition for their focus on specific genetic conditions. Genetic etiologies provided a distinct mode of distinguishing patient populations, and recognition of the diverse outcomes across a single genotype made the idea of "severity" less salient. In 1992, ABMS granted medical geneticists their own medical specialty board—akin to ABP and ABPN. After this, medical geneticists enjoyed a level of recognition and prestige that was never available to developmental disabilities specialists in pediatrics or neurology, which may have afforded some with greater independence to promote new views on disability.[99]

Down syndrome, the most prevalent developmental disability with a discrete genetic cause, was a common specialty area for many late twentieth-century medical geneticists and some pediatricians. Notably, Down syndrome did not fit neatly into either the NDD or DBP subspecialty domain—the condition was not listed among Capute's spectrum of developmental disabilities and was rarely addressed by behavioral pediatricians. Various professional pathways led pediatricians to focus on Down syndrome. During the late 1960s, pediatrician Siegfried Pueschel founded the Boston Children's Hospital Down Syndrome Program, just a few years after his son Christian was born with the condition (chapter 2). A decade later, when Pueschel left to become the director of the Child Development Center at Brown University, his pediatrics colleague Allen Crocker took over primary responsibility for the Down Syndrome Program.[100]

Crocker began his career in pediatrics during the 1950s, working under Sidney Farber at Boston Children's Hospital on rare metabolic conditions like Tay-Sachs disease. When federal funding became available in the 1960s to construct University Affiliated Facilities on mental retardation, Crocker was one of the program's first grantees. He became the founding director of the Boston Children's Hospital Development Evaluation Center in 1967. Crocker later stated that he had been "lucky enough to get caught up in [the Down syndrome] Movement," which was being driven by parent advocates and government investments in the 1960s and '70s (chapter 2). He quickly realized that disabled children were not being treated as "full citizens" and became active in sociopolitical advocacy that worked toward radical changes.[101] Reflecting on Crocker's accomplishments, pediatric medical geneticist Brian Skotko, who trained with him in the 2000s, said, "Parents fight fewer battles because Allen [Crocker] tore down walls."[102]

Skotko noted that, over time, Crocker "fell in love" with the unique personalities of children with Down syndrome and openly celebrated their strengths and accomplishments.[103] He may have been one of the first physicians to unreservedly congratulate parents on the birth of their new child—who happened to have Down syndrome. While Crocker engaged in and valued biomedical research on Down syndrome, as he grew older he became unabashedly more humanistic and political in his orientation. He focused on the need to "get our societal house in order in terms of humans of different kinds all living together in mutual happiness."[104] As part of this, Crocker was a highly regarded member of the Massachusetts Down Syndrome Congress. He also edited *Bus Girl*, a book of poems by Gretchen Josephson, who had Down syndrome. Crocker's perspective and approaches brought a more light-hearted and accepting tone to the area of developmental disabilities, even as he battled to make significant political headway.

During the 1980s, Crocker was also a prominent member of the Society for Behavioral Pediatrics, serving as its president in 1987–1988. In this role, Crocker pushed for increased political engagement by SBP and created an ad hoc Social Concerns Committee to help mobilize advocacy for children and raise societal consciousness about the challenges young people faced.[105] While Crocker was a highly regarded leader in the DBP field, he never got involved in the subspecialty push. During his time as SBP president, it was not yet a major topic of discussion. Crocker's farewell remarks as president, delivered in 1988, were notable for their atypical focus and revealed his unique interests and approach. Instead of talking about research, identity, or other professional concerns, Crocker chose to read aloud a number of poems—for children, about children, and by children. As he explained it, "There is a lot of behavioral pediatrics in children's poems, and there are a lot of children's poems inside all of us behavioral pediatricians."[106] For Crocker, poetry was a way of breaking down barriers between professional and patient perspectives. Reading poetry also encouraged pediatricians to remember what it was like to be a child and how they learned about and engaged in the world as a young person.

Crocker did contribute significantly to the DBP field. He was a founding coeditor, along with Melvin Levine and William Carey, of the area's first and most prominent textbook, *Developmental-Behavioral Pediatrics* (1983). Particularly notable in this book was the last chapter, "The Right to Be Different." In it, the editors argued that the legal victories of the 1960s and '70s had not yet been matched by sufficient advances in the acceptance of "very different" children in the social realm. While much of the thrust in the clinical professions was to make these children more "normal," the editors called for celebrating the value of human diversity, including disability. As Levine, Carey, and Crocker put it in the textbook's second edition, published in 1992, "Those most familiar with human variation . . . ultimately become captivated by the commonality of values and continuum of contribution."[107]

"The Right to be Different" chapter was initially Levine's idea, but it is clear that Crocker added significantly to its framing and message, especially when it came to promoting equal rights, optimism, and appreciation for children with "severe" disabilities. Crocker had previously written about the tendency of professionals to shy away from significantly disabled children. He presented the alternate view that all humans, no matter their level of disability, could achieve and appreciate their mastery of certain tasks. There was always the opportunity for clinicians to be enthralled by the accomplishments of their patients. Crocker was well ahead of his time among clinicians in this push to honor and celebrate difference in the realm of disability.[108] His perspectives and efforts aimed to encourage the DBP field to actively include in their domain children with more "severe" developmental disabilities, while also adopting more optimistic and accepting narratives of developmental disabilities than what was commonplace in NDD or DBP.

Crocker's dedication and efforts offered an excellent model for taking up and promoting more positive, inclusive, and sociopolitical views of people with developmental disabilities. He unapologetically engaged in community and political advocacy, while espousing celebratory narratives of disability among his patients and colleagues. Crocker's approaches broke with dominant postwar training models in genetic counseling and other clinical professionals, which encouraged "neutral" biomedical explanations, "nondirective" patient counseling, and maintaining "professional distance" from families' experiences.[109] In the next chapter, I examine many genetic counselors' reluctance toward clinical engagement and political advocacy that directly encouraged more optimistic and accepting views of Down syndrome and other developmental disabilities. As I explore, in the 2010s, new political forces began to reveal and undermine some of the core interests that genetic counselors and disability advocates shared.

6

Keeping the Conversation Open

Genetic Counseling, Disability,

and Selective Abortion

In 1992, epidemiologist Abby Lippman and pediatrician Benjamin Wilfond powerfully argued in their article "Twice-Told Tales: Stories about Genetic Disorders" that two distinct narratives of Down syndrome were being presented in the prenatal versus the postnatal contexts. Their evidence was based on an informal survey of the clinical literature provided after a Down syndrome diagnosis. Lippman and Wilfond found that "the *before*-birth information is largely negative, focusing on technical matters and describing the array of potential medical complications and physical limitations that may occur in children with the condition, while *after*-birth information tends to be more positive, focusing on compensating aspects of the condition, highlighting the availability of medical and social resources, and setting hope for the future."[1] Behind these narratives, they suggested, were distinct messages about what should be done in response to a Down syndrome diagnosis—with a clear preference for prevention via selective abortion. While Lippman and Wilfond acknowledged that no educational materials were truly neutral, they argued that the existence of such different messages for the same condition raised important questions about whether clinicians should be providing more balanced narratives.

As prenatal diagnosis became widespread in the United States after 1975, the master's level field of genetic counseling grew alongside it. In the prenatal context, genetic counselors provided information about testing, risks, and biomedical conditions and helped their patients to make reproductive choices that best fit with their personal values and goals. The field actively sought to distance its identity and ambitions from those of eugenicists, who wanted to "improve" society and its gene pool by encouraging or enforcing certain reproductive decisions. Instead, genetic counselors embraced "non-directive" practices, while avoiding any outward claims of pursuing societal end goals, like the widespread prevention of genetic conditions.[2]

Even though prenatal genetic counselors prioritized individual choices, they worked within an infrastructure that was largely justified by the assumption that prenatal testing and selective abortion would reduce the incidence of disability and save society money.[3] After a diagnosis of developmental disabilities, couples faced difficult decisions. Most chose abortion. These persistent outcomes led many disability advocates to suggest that genetic counselors were too often characterizing life with disabilities as tragic and hopeless. Instead, advocates argued that genetic counselors had a responsibility to acknowledge and address the broader impacts of selective abortion on societal perceptions of the nature and acceptability of life with disabilities.

Confronted with critiques from disability advocates, most genetic counselors remained focused on facilitating the independent choices of pregnant women. Genetic counselors were wary of shifts in practice that might alter their patients' reproductive decision-making—even when this involved counteracting the overly negative and misinformed perceptions of disabled people that many held. Ultimately, there was little hope for a resolution that would adequately address the serious concerns of disability advocates about selective abortion without disrupting genetic counselors' fundamental commitment to respecting reproductive choice. In this chapter, I argue that even with no likely pathway to consensus, there was still value in ongoing debates and open dialogues between disability advocates and genetic counselors. In a field with short training programs (two years), the regular rekindling of discussions about genetic counselors' relationships and responsibilities to disabled people helped to prevent these issues from consistently being overshadowed by the latest biomedical innovations and testing options.

This chapter explores disability self-advocates' direct and influential role, during the 1990s and 2000s, in pushing genetic counselors to have greater awareness and engagement with more positive, inclusive, and sociopolitical perspectives on disability, as well as concerns about disability discrimination and oppression. Self-advocates developed personal relationships with genetic counselors, actively participated in the field's conferences, and helped to shape the training and perceptions of some genetic counseling trainees. At the same time, the National Society of Genetic Counselors (NSGC) largely overlooked or dismissed the concerns of disability self-advocates and a small contingent of likeminded genetic counselors. Leaders in the field remained focused on highlighting genetic counselors' primary professional role as patient educators and facilitators of reproductive choice in clinical settings and their identity as biomedical experts and sociopolitical advocates for reproductive autonomy and access to abortion.

During the 2010s, more genetic counselors began to appreciate that they and disability self-advocates faced common obstacles in achieving a shared ambition to bring about more fully informed choices during pregnancy. Legislative efforts by pro-life partisans interfered with efforts to make standardized and comprehensive information about disabilities available to all pregnant couples and families. Multiple US states also outlawed selective abortion for Down syndrome and other conditions—effectively removing the purpose and opportunity for genetic counselors to engage patients in substantive conversations about disability. These discussions, before or during prenatal diagnosis, were an important entry point for countering pessimistic assumptions and reached many people who would never know a disabled person. Also, as the political landscape for prenatal diagnosis was shifting, genetic counselors were moving into new niches. By 2020, only 37 percent worked in prenatal settings, whereas 52 percent did cancer counseling.[4]

In this chapter, I examine multiple successful efforts to enhance disability advocacy among genetic counselors, as well as various biomedical, professional, and political barriers to more universal moves in this direction. Ultimately, it was not more diverse information—which included positive and accepting narratives of disability—that undermined patients' autonomous decision-making in the prenatal context. Rather, it was legal, professional, and technological factors that undermined choice and the important opportunity to consider one's alternatives.

Genetic Counselors and Abortion Rights Advocacy

During the 1980s, as amniocentesis became more prevalent in the United States, genetic counselors were increasingly involved and associated with prenatal diagnosis. In 1981, 61 percent of genetic counselors reported that prenatal services were part of their professional responsibilities. A decade later, half of genetic counselors reported that they engaged exclusively in prenatal practice, and another 25 percent listed a combination of prenatal and pediatric counseling.[5] At the same time, abortion had become a more fraught political issue. After Ronald Reagan's election to the US presidency in 1980 on a pro-life platform, leaders in genetic counseling expressed concern about continued abortion access. Retiring NSGC President Beverly Rolnick warned colleagues, "Congressional efforts to define when life begins and to restrict accessibility to abortion affect public perception and support of certain types of genetic services, especially prenatal diagnosis."[6]

Four years later, NSGC cofounder Judith Widmann noted genetic counselors' significant professional interest in protecting abortion rights and argued, "I would like the NSGC itself to take a firm stand on the side of prochoice while it can still do so. It would be unthinkable to have this right taken away while NSGC did nothing."[7] A subsequent member survey found that 93 percent favored NSGC becoming officially engaged in pro-choice activities.[8] NSGC soon developed relationships with the National Abortion Rights Action League, Planned Parenthood, and the Religious Coalition for Abortion Rights. The Society's professional newsletter, *Perspectives in Genetic Counseling*, also started a new Legislative Briefs section, which was prominently displayed on its back page immediately above the recipient's address. Among other topics, this section highlighted and encouraged participation in pro-choice marches and signature drives.

Just a few NSGC members opposed the Society's engagement in pro-choice activities. One genetic counselor warned that NSGC's public positions risked "damaging the reputation of the organization collectively and of its members individually. . . . [T]he uneducated public may be confused by these messages and misconstrue 'pro-choice' to 'pro-abortion.'" Vivian Weinblatt, the chair of NSGC's Social Issues Committee pushed back, stating that genetic counselors had a responsibility to "lobby for our patients' rights to all options. When state legislatures limit availability of abortion, we are less able to provide a full range of options to our patients. . . . Anything less is shirking our ethical responsibility as patient advocates."[9] Weinblatt believed that defending abortion access was central to genetic counselors' professional role and identity.

Most late twentieth-century genetic counselors avoided sociopolitical advocacy activities outside of the clinic (chapter 3), so the field's active and broad-based engagement with the hot button issue of abortion is particularly notable. Pro-choice advocacy fit comfortably with genetic counselors' strong commitment to facilitating autonomous reproductive decision-making. However, from the perspective of disability self-advocates, many of who were strongly pro-choice themselves, genetic counselors' prominent investment in defending abortion rights without similar support for disability rights and perspectives reflected their indifference toward the oppressive impacts of selective abortion on societal perceptions of disabled people.

Indeed, while NSGC took an official position on abortion rights in 1986, it did not release a position statement on disability until 2011. During the intervening quarter century, some disability self-advocates began actively targeting their critical messages about prenatal diagnosis and selective abortion to genetic counselors, with the hope that influencing the field could help to achieve larger societal changes in this area. Through their efforts, disability advocates succeeded in encouraging open dialogues with some genetic counselors and influencing some training programs' engagement with the perspectives and experiences of disabled people. Into the 2000s, however, these achievements remained limited and were largely not institutionalized by NSGC.

Engaging with Disability Perspectives

Adrienne Asch influenced numerous genetic counselors and medical geneticists during the 1990s. She was a social psychologist and bioethicist, who became blind soon after birth and was an outspoken disability and women's self-advocate. In 1993, Asch wrote about "subtle and not-so-subtle bias against disabled people by some geneticists who do the science and by some genetic counselors who translate science to the public. . . . Our discomfort arises out of the knowledge that when information about life with disability is described at all, it usually is a description filled with gloom and tragedy."[10] Many clinical professionals were struck by Asch's fierce independence, strongly defended beliefs, incisive mentorship, and blunt personality. Over her career, Asch greatly influenced—and memorably chastised—numerous clinicians for their ableist understandings and actions. She introduced to the attention of many clinical thought leaders the overlooked, discriminatory impacts of genetics, prenatal testing, and everyday language on disabled people—and inspired them to work toward change in their field.

Disability advocates' perceptions that many genetic counselors held and expressed strongly negative views of people with disabilities were backed by research. In 1988, W. Carl Cooley, a pediatrician whose daughter Sarah had Down syndrome, videotaped a discussion he had with ten other parents of children with Down syndrome. Cooley showed the recording to mothers of children with Down syndrome, obstetric nurses, and genetic counselors. Most of the mothers reacted positively to the video, and the nurses were supportive of its clinical value. However, the great majority of the genetic counselors viewed the video as inaccurate and useless because they felt that it had glossed over important clinical details. Nearly half of the genetic counselors surveyed also stated that they would personally choose abortion for Down syndrome.[11]

Self-advocate Marsha Saxton was another vocal critic of genetic counseling, based in part on her own experiences. She recalled a genetic counseling session from the early 1980s:

> The genetic counselor said to me, "If I had known 'spina bifidas' could turn out as well as you, then I would not have recommended selective abortion." [Saxton replied to the counselor,] "I guess you mean that as a compliment, but that is a weird thing to say to me. I may be privileged as a less disabled version of this, but I have many friends with spina bifida who are more disabled than I am. I think that their lives are worth living and that they're wonderful people."[12]

Saxton initially trained in speech pathology but was disenchanted by the health care system and eventually left the field to become a disability and women's rights advocate in Boston. In 1984, she proposed, "Genetics professionals should take responsibility to learn about and teach more accurate pictures of disability. They need to examine their own values and fears about disability, and how these can influence their work. Ideally this process would begin early in the training programs."[13]

During the early 1990s, as part of her PhD dissertation research, Saxton brought her vision to fruition of encouraging a deeper awareness and engagement with disability perspectives among genetic counseling students. She developed a working relationship with the newly formed genetic counseling training program at Brandeis University and recruited students to participate in her study. Drawing on her connections with the disability advocacy community in Boston, she also recruited adults with physical disabilities to participate. Each community member was paired with a genetic counseling student—they met together three times in community locations and got to know one another on a personal level. Such engagement was rare in training programs. Most of the genetic counseling students had otherwise only interacted with disabled adults in clinical settings, if at all. In follow-up interviews with the students, Saxton found that their views of disability were powerfully affected toward an understanding that disability was strongly shaped by social context, that it did not imply a tragic life, and that they could easily be friends or colleagues with disabled adults. Although Saxton soon left for a position in California, her engagement model continued to be used at Brandeis for a decade.[14]

Notably, the Brandeis program stood out from most other genetic counseling training programs in the 1990s because of its significant efforts to engage with the perspectives and experiences of people in the disability community. Judith Tsipis, a PhD biologist, founded the program in 1992. Her son Andreas had disabilities related to Canavan disease, a neurological condition.[15] Although not a trained genetic counselor herself, Tsipis was committed to developing and leading a training curriculum that would actively address disability issues throughout. This included an annual seminar, in which disabled adults with genetic conditions were invited to engage students about their experiences, and a Family Pals program, where genetic counseling trainees learned firsthand about the joys and challenges of raising a disabled child through close engagement and social activities with disabled children and families.[16]

A diverse advisory board oversaw the Brandeis training program. Its members included Saxton and Irving Kenneth Zola, another prominent disability scholar and self-advocate. Zola was a medical sociologist at Brandeis and had physical disabilities from polio and a later car accident. In the early 1980s he began writing about his experiences as a disabled person in academia and advocating for himself; he helped to establish the discipline of disability studies, as well as the journal *Disability Studies Quarterly*.[17] While other genetic counseling programs followed Tsipis's lead over the next three decades, in adding significantly more classroom and experiential content related to disability, Brandeis was one of just a few programs in the 1990s to demonstrate how genetic counseling could place disability awareness and advocacy at its core rather than at the periphery of training and practice (chapter 3). Historian Alexandra Stern has argued that more widespread adoption of Brandeis's model could help the genetic counseling field to finally overcome the long-standing practice of elevating reproductive autonomy above all else.[18]

Outside of her dissertation work, Saxton also organized a disability dialogue session in 1996 involving 40 genetic counselors, a number of disability scholars and advocates, and women who had personal experiences with prenatal diagnosis and selective abortion. It was an opportunity to bring new disability narratives to genetic counselors at a later stage of their careers. Previous forums on these topics had been set up as bioethics debates, but Saxton designed a listening session focused on personal narratives about continuing or ending pregnancies after prenatal testing.[19] Five genetic counselors who attended later reported in the *Perspectives* newsletter: "We left the meeting feeling that bonds were formed, bridges built and prejudices challenged—well demonstrated by one participant's comment: 'I was expecting to confront narrow-minded disability-phobic genetic professionals—what a surprise to meet so many professionals who turned my stereotypes around.'"[20] As Saxton had intended, personal conversations helped genetic counselors and disability self-advocates to identify common experiences, concerns, and goals related to prenatal testing and disability discrimination.

Another landmark collaborative gathering to discuss the intersection of prenatal diagnosis and disability rights began around the same time. Erik Parens of the Hastings Center Bioethics Research Institute in New York had organized this multiyear series of meetings. Parens brought together physicians, genetic counselors, ethicists, and disability self-advocates with the goal of encouraging open engagement, reducing long-standing tensions, and seeking consensus. Saxton and Asch participated, along with genetic counselor Barbara Biesecker (chapter 3) and Benjamin Wilfond, a pediatrician and bioethics scholar. Asch presented her view that selective abortion for disabilities was an expressive form of discrimination, which conveyed the message that life with a disability was tragic and unacceptable. She argued, "As with discrimination more generally, with prenatal diagnosis, a single trait stands in for the whole, the trait obliterates the whole. With both discrimination and prenatal diagnosis, nobody finds out about the rest."[21] Further, Parens and Asch noted, such views extended to people who possessed the undesired trait, leading to oppressive attitudes, low expectations, and poor supports for disabled people.[22]

Notably, Saxton and Asch each held strongly pro-choice views on abortion, and neither was fundamentally opposed to prenatal testing. As Saxton put it, "In a different world, I wouldn't have a problem with prenatal diagnosis. But within the context of existing oppression, acts that would otherwise NOT be considered oppressive become oppressive acts within that context."[23] Saxton and Asch both believed that disabled people's challenges were not rooted in prenatal testing itself but rather in the society where it took place.

Asch stated, "I have never said . . . that testing should be outlawed for any reason for any condition. . . . Some effort to help women obtain information about life with disability is important, and until it happens, women will draw on tests in large part unknowingly and inappropriately." In this sense, Saxton and Asch agreed with most genetic counselors that providing adequate information was the best path forward. However, this had to include positive narratives of disability as well, or as Asch suggested, at least had to present disability as one among the many unique characteristics of an individual.[24]

One major topic of discussion at the Hastings meeting was whether bioethicists could and should "draw lines" to help delineate ethically, socially, or medically appropriate uses of prenatal testing. The participants debated the implications and potential approaches to determining which conditions were sufficiently "severe" to justify prenatal diagnosis and selective abortion. Some bioethicists in attendance at Hastings, including Jeffrey Botkin, supported developing line-drawing logics and efforts to distinguish "severe" disabilities. Whereas, Asch, Wilfond, and Dorothy Wertz argued that the severity of disabilities was both variable and rooted in constructed value judgments. As they noted, every family interpreted and handled their child's disability differently, meaning that no universal lines could be drawn.[25] Which instances of disability counted as "severe" would always be a matter of interpretation. At the same time, the practice of labeling particular disabilities as "severe" helped to facilitate or justify discriminatory policies, treatments, or (non)interventions—including selective abortion, starvation, electroshock, presumed illiteracy, and deferral to another medical subspecialty (chapters 2, 4, and 5).

After five meetings, held over two years, no universal consensus was achieved by the Hastings meeting participants. One area of general accord was that genetic counselors and other clinicians could engage their patients in better-informed prenatal decision-making by providing them with more carefully balanced information, which included families' challenges as well as their positive experiences. Going further, the participants stated, "If genetics professionals and obstetrical providers are to help individuals make truly informed decisions, then they, like everybody else in the 'majority' community must identify and overcome biases against people with disabilities." Achieving this would involve better education for clinical professionals who provided prenatal counseling. Saxton's dissertation work at Brandeis was an important model for this. Patient education needed to be improved as well and begin before any prenatal testing was performed. Such engagement would help couples reflect on their views of disability and on what it would mean for them to have a disabled child, and then to consider their goals for testing.[26]

The Hastings meetings had a transformative impact on the perspectives of some clinicians. Biesecker recalled that the gatherings were among the best experiences of her career. She later invited Asch to engage with genetic counselors in other settings, including by presenting and commenting—often forcefully—at NSGC conferences. Medical geneticist John Carey recounted having been invited to Hastings meetings and said that he had "always regretted" turning down the opportunity. Nonetheless, Carey got to know Asch and very much admired her. He recalled telling Asch about how bad he had felt as a resident in pediatrics when, for the first time, he needed give a Down syndrome diagnosis—but was very poorly prepared to do so (chapter 2). Her response was etched in this memory; she said, "You should have felt bad." Asch, he recounted, drew his attention to what he didn't know about the experiences of disabled people, and she inspired him to want to understand more.[27]

Wilfond characterized the Hastings meetings as "more than an academic exercise. It was personally meaningful, with a genuine and respectful level of interest, exploration, and engagement." He credited Parens for bringing together people with diverse views and for encouraging meaningful conversations about their disagreements rather than consensus.[28] As a pediatrician and bioethics scholar, Wilfond challenged his clinical colleagues' overly negative and functionally oriented interpretations of disability. Like Robert Cooke, Wilfond sought to remind clinicians that their perspectives on "suffering" were socially constructed and specific to their own experiences (chapter 2). In the clinic, Wilfond supported parents' choices to keep their "severely" disabled children on ventilators, sometimes to the frustration of his colleagues who recommended discontinuing intervention. He recounted such an experience in a 2014 *Pediatrics* article, in which he argued that clinicians and bioethicists needed to consider the capacity of children to form relationships with people, and how their families valued these relationships, in making their pronouncements about whether life-sustaining interventions should be continued.[29]

Collaborative gatherings, like Saxton's disability dialogues and the Hastings Center meetings, helped to increase engagement, understanding, and trust between disability self-advocates and some genetic counselors. Saxton had initially assumed that genetic counselors would have significant influence in the genetic testing arena, but over time came to appreciate that they, like disability self-advocates, were often marginalized by PhD geneticists and physicians. In particular, she pointed to her participation on the National Institutes of Health (NIH) Ethical, Legal, and Social Implications (ELSI) of the Human Genome Project (HGP) working group, noting, "We were tokenized as these marginal voices because they had to pretend that they were including the workers in the field, like the genetic counselors, and the consumers of genetic testing and the disability community, but there was no real effort to listen to what we were saying."[30] Genetic counselors were in a position to influence individual women's perspectives on prenatal diagnosis and disabilities, but counselors were largely excluded from scientific, clinical, and institutional decisions about developing, marketing, and offering new genetic tests.

As director of the joint Johns Hopkins / NIH genetic counseling training program, Biesecker also had an insider's perspective on the limitations that genetic counselors faced. She criticized how new prenatal tests were too often introduced with little serious social or ethical consideration. At NIH, Biesecker noted, any attempt at writing testing guidelines was dismissed, even when the test screened for "what might be considered normal variation in a fetus." She told the Hastings Center meeting participants, "The prevailing attitude around the institution [is] . . . since we can not get consensus on genetic issues, do not even bother trying. Any test is acceptable, except for sex." These geneticists, she felt, had "no sense of responsibility" for the availability of specific prenatal tests, how patients used them, or the tests' broader societal impacts.[31]

Reflecting on genetic counselors' perspectives and responsibilities within this context of unrestrained testing, Biesecker and Lori Hamby later argued, "Without realizing it, many counselors may carry an overly 'medicalized' view of genetic and nongenetic disabilities. . . . [T]o help give women exploring the option of prenatal testing a true vision of the experience of having a child with a disability, a prenatal counselor should have experience with people across the lifespan who are living with such circumstances."[32] Such recognition and reform in genetic counseling practice was a long-standing goal of Saxton, Asch, and other self-advocates. Biesecker spoke for a small but growing contingent of genetic counselors who incorporated these views into their approaches and training programs (chapter 3). Still, as the scope of prenatal testing expanded in the 1990s and 2000s, conflicts and tensions continued among genetic counselors and disability advocates.

NSGC and Disability Advocacy

Disability scholars powerfully influenced a small contingent of genetic counselors during the 1990s. These practitioners understood that many of their colleagues were better prepared to provide pathological descriptions of disabilities than more positive and accepting narratives. Indeed, with the exception of a few unique training programs (chapter 3), most genetic counselors rarely engaged with real world disability viewpoints. Genetic counselor Campbell Brasington recalled, "My graduate training [during the late 1980s] taught me to maintain a 'professional distance.' But the most rewarding and meaningful aspect of my work has been the relationships I've developed working *together* with families and people with Down syndrome over the years" (emphasis in original).[33] Most genetic counselors—as students or while in practice in prenatal settings—never benefited from these relationships. With their professional roles, identity, and approaches already established, it also seemed unlikely that many would reexamine how they facilitated autonomous reproductive choices.

Looking to the institutional level, NSGC had historically built alliances with biotechnology companies and abortion providers, while overlooking the concerns of disability self-advocates about prenatal diagnosis. The major financial supporters of NSGC's *Perspectives* newsletter during the 1990s and 2000s were Integrated Genetics—a company that sold prenatal tests—and Women's Health Care Services—a late-term abortion provider. Such organizations also had a major presence at conferences. Genetic counselor Kathryn Peters recalled an NSGC meeting in the late 1990s: "It hit me how completely bizarre of an organization we are that we have abortion service providers directly across from . . . [disability] groups, whose mission, on some level, is to give support to people who are continuing pregnancies, and allow people to accept the idea that it is not so bad, that I can live with this."[34] Professional conflicts between facilitating reproductive autonomy and supporting disabled people were prominently on display at genetic counseling conferences and in the field's publications. Peters did not feel that NSGC acknowledged any responsibility to recognize and balance these competing interests.

Peters was affiliated with the joint Johns Hopkins / NIH genetic counseling program and brought her observations and concerns to Biesecker. Together, they helped to develop a journal article presenting their perspectives on genetic counseling's uneven commitment to prenatal diagnosis versus disability advocacy. Anne Madeo, another genetic counselor at NIH, became the lead author. Together, the five coauthors held a wide spectrum of views on the legality and uptake of abortion. They wrote,

> The NSGC's prominent sponsorships by late-term abortion providers appear to support concerns of disability advocates that genetic counselors value abortion rights over the worth of the lives of those affected by disabling conditions. . . . The NSGC has a professional obligation to publically support reproductive freedoms for clients, just as it should publically support the needs of disabled clients. If counselors do not speak up on behalf of clients who choose *not* to terminate a pregnancy, then who will? If counselors do not also speak up on behalf of clients with disabilities, then who will?[35]

Further, they explained that genetic testing companies and abortion providers had clear financial advantages over disability advocacy groups for advertising. What, they asked, was NSGC doing to provide a counterweight to these interest groups' monetary largess and greater prominence to ensure that the voices and views of disability advocates were also visibly displayed for, and known by, NSGC members?

Madeo and colleagues' article, which was published in 2011, led to renewed discussion about the genetic counseling profession's perceptions of and responsibilities to disabled people. The publication also played a major part in pushing NSGC to adopt that same year its first official position statement on people with disabilities. Nonetheless, NSGC leaders responded defensively to the article's arguments, noting,

> In their subjective commentary, Madeo et al. imply that discussing reproductive choices with clients and describing medical aspects of certain diagnoses in some way devalues people with disabilities. We concur that genetic counselors . . . must not favor, or even appear to favor, one group over another. The NSGC contends that, more than other professionals, genetic counselors have the unique ability to address all sides of these complex issues.[36]

Not surprisingly, the field's leaders highlighted their preferred characterization of genetic counselors' distinctive strengths—to maintain neutrality and see issues from all sides. It is notable, however, that they did so while

dismissing their own colleagues' observations and representing their perspectives as merely "subjective."

Patricia Bauer, a journalist whose daughter Margaret had Down syndrome, challenged the idea that genetic counselors could or should try to be
neutral. She wrote,

> I worry that professionals within the prenatal testing world, often without even
> being aware of it, are shading their messages in such a way as to transform the
> right to terminate into something that feels more like an obligation to termi-
> nate. . . . I don't think physicians and genetic counselors are sending this mes-
> sage deliberately. But, regardless of intent, the effect is the same. These sublim-
> inal messages support a climate in which disability discrimination can flourish
> unchallenged.[37]

Arguing, as NSGC did, that genetic counselors were uniquely able to address
all sides of the issue was not that same as taking seriously the need for
greater awareness of potential harms.

Genetic counselor Robert Resta offered a reflective response from within
the profession. He challenged some of the defensiveness of genetic counselors toward the article's arguments, noting, "The natural reaction to criticism
is 'Wait a minute. We are non-directive about abortion, support everyone's
autonomy and reproductive rights, and do our best to provide unbiased
information.'" He then acknowledged that "a complicated and controversial
counseling topic has been raised; this is an opportunity to explore it. . . .
[I]f we open our minds and try to see past our deeply ingrained biases we
will grow as individuals and as a profession."[38] While it was natural and stra-
tegic to react defensively to criticism from within the field, Resta—in line with
Bauer and others—sought to reinforce the value of critical self-reflection
among genetic counselors.

Over the next couple of years, a few more articles were published in the
genetic counseling literature on disability-related topics, including a special
issue of the *Journal of Genetic Counseling* on developmental disabilities.[39]
Genetic counselor Melissa Lenihan described her own experiences as the
mother of a disabled child and encouraged more engagement with disability
issues in the profession. She wrote,

> I think it would behoove us as genetic counselors to step back from the medical
> model . . . and move towards a more humanistic approach. The seeming discon-

nect for genetic counselors between supporting patients who choose to terminate an affected pregnancy while purporting to simultaneously support the disability community is something that I am living on a daily basis. I have to admit
it is at times uncomfortable.[40]

Lenihan encouraged her colleagues to engage with their patients' fears
about disability, as well as their own, to help facilitate a more truly informed
decision-making process.

Another article examined 93 transcripts from genetic counseling sessions conducted in 2003–2004. It found that social aspects of disability were
only discussed in 27 percent of sessions and that patients were asked about
their own personal experiences with disability just 38 percent of the time.
Further, the authors directly engaged with disability advocacy critiques of
prenatal diagnosis, suggesting that genetic counselors should do more to
directly investigate patients' knowledge and perceptions of disability and
recommending that this begin earlier in the testing process.[41]

While various articles, blog posts, and master's theses engaged and
responded to Madeo and colleague's 2011 paper over the next three years,
there was little evidence of any significant changes in NSGC or the broader
field's approaches to disability during this period.[42] The official NSGC statement on disability, which was initially published in response to Madeo's
article, called for celebrating each individual's value and diversity and avoiding defining people by a single characteristic. NSGC also acknowledged,
"Technological advancements in genetics may potentially benefit individuals
with disabilities; however, they may also cause harm or stigmatize. Policies
should be enacted around these technologies to ensure safeguards protect
the rights of those with physical, cognitive, or psychiatric differences and
their families."[43]

Madeo felt that NSGC's statement "says all the right things without suggesting that they are going to do a single thing. . . . I am not convinced that
they are doing anything differently that actually suggests they are trying to
make any changes."[44] NSGC did not choose to directly engage with the professional conflicts that arose at the intersection of prenatal testing and disability advocacy. Rather, the Society's responses to these concerns, even when
expressed by its own members, were largely defensive and rhetorical. As
genetic counselor Laura Hercher put it, NSGC fell back on their favored narrative that "genetic counselors are trained good-doers," who work within the

medical context to protect patients' interests.[45] Many genetic counselors believed that they were already doing their part on disability advocacy through their professional role as clinically based advocates for individual patients and families. Some genetic counselors, though, believed that their field could have a unique part to play in bringing people together and encouraging open and productive conversations across professional and ideological divides.

Seeking Consensus on Prenatal Testing

Serious consideration of disability perspectives in genetic counseling waxed and waned during the first decades of the twenty-first century. In 2007, discussion of the social impacts of prenatal testing came back to the foreground when the American College of Obstetricians and Gynecologists (ACOG) announced a major policy change—recommending that all women, independent of age or other risk factors, should be offered prenatal testing for various detectable conditions, including Down syndrome. Amniocentesis had always been considered to pose some risk of miscarriage but was now deemed safe enough for all pregnancies.[46] This policy change was likely to expand the number and range of women who underwent testing and chose selective abortion, and it reenflamed tensions between clinical and disability advocacy communities.

The next year Janice Edwards, the director of the University of South Carolina genetic counseling training program, organized a gathering of representatives from various clinical and disability advocacy communities to discuss prenatal testing. She strongly believed that somebody needed "to get these people together to talk to each other because they do not understand each other's intentions."[47] Edwards invited genetic counselor Campbell Brasington to help organize the conference. As a trainee at the University of South Carolina in the late 1980s, Brasington had been assigned to work with a Down syndrome support group. The experience had inspired her long-term commitment to disability engagement and advocacy. Brasington found that, as a genetic counselor, disability advocacy groups did not always warmly welcome her. She recalled, "Just out of graduate school, I started attending meetings of our local Down syndrome support group. I remember the first meeting I went to, one parent came up to me and said accusingly, 'What are you doing here? You're a genetic counselor!!' as if all we did was perform prenatal diagnosis and terminate pregnancies of babies with Down syndrome."[48]

Such tensions were common in the 1990s and 2000s; Edwards and Brasington believed open dialogues could help.

With assistance from her colleague Anthony Gregg, an obstetrician and medical geneticist, Edwards organized a consensus conference in 2008, which was attended by representatives of multiple professional and advocacy groups, including ACOG, NSGC, the American College of Medical Genetics (ACMG), National Down Syndrome Society (NDSS), and National Down Syndrome Congress (NDSC). Prominent advocate Madeline Will, whose son Jon has Down syndrome, represented NDSS. Edwards recounted that she was initially nervous to engage with Will but found that their conversations quickly became easy and productive.

The consensus conference also began with trepidation on all sides. Representatives from advocacy groups came with assumptions about the aims of clinicians. ACOG participants were uneasy due to frequent picketing by parent groups after their 2007 policy change. Hearing personal stories from all sides about experiences with caring for children with Down syndrome helped the participants to build rapport and move forward on identifying areas of agreement.[49]

Edwards's consensus conference produced a list of six agreed-upon misconceptions about prenatal testing, which included the misperception that obstetricians "recommend prenatal tests to reduce the number of individuals in society who have birth defects and genetic conditions" and "to decrease the number of births of children with Down syndrome." The participants also established that NDSS and NDSC were not pro-life organizations and that genetic counselors did not influence parents to accept pregnancy termination.[50] Notably, each consensus point was largely defensive—the participants agreed that their aims were misunderstood. Genetic counselors reemphasized their role and identity as educators and facilitators of choice—not promoters of abortion. They did not highlight a parallel identity as disability advocates.

Nothing in the consensus document acknowledged the critiques of disability self-advocates that prenatal diagnosis and selective abortion had discriminatory and oppressive impacts on disabled people. Indeed, no disability self-advocates were invited or selected to attend, even by the disability advocacy organizations. Brasington, who participated as an NSGC representative, later suggested that the group was not yet ready to address these issues. She explained, "At that time, there was still some distrust with each other: like what's your real agenda, or how am I going to be portrayed after this? . . . There were lots of other areas we could have addressed . . . [but] we did not have the time or the relationships yet to do that." Edwards noted that the goal of the meeting was to get professional and advocacy organizations talking and that their common concern was prenatal testing—not social perceptions of disability.[51] However, these two issues were unavoidably linked, since patient choices concerning prenatal testing and selective abortion were very much influenced by pessimistic clinical and societal narratives of disability. While the consensus conference succeeded in opening up new lines of communication, it was primarily a forum in which clinical and advocacy professionals discussed their own concerns, more so than those of disabled people.

Importantly, the University of South Carolina consensus group was a nucleus for ongoing collaboration among clinicians and professional disability advocates over the coming years. A number of the participants contributed to developing a "gold standard" information packet to be distributed to *all* families upon receiving a prenatal or pediatric Down syndrome diagnosis. This booklet had the potential to become the universal resource that Abby Lippman and Benjamin Wilfond had called for, nearly two decades earlier, in their "Twice Told Tales" article.

Medical geneticist Brian Skotko, whose sister Kristin has Down syndrome, was a leader in the push to establish and promote more optimistic guidelines for presenting diagnoses to families.[52] Skotko highlighted that participants in the effort, which began in 2008, all agreed that, "the information needed to be honest, balanced, and real in order to be believable and used."[53] The booklet would also have to satisfy a wide range of interest groups, including obstetricians, genetic counselors, medical geneticists, and disability advocacy organizations. For a variety of professional and political reasons, this proved to be a more difficult challenge than anticipated.

Barriers to Standardized Information

In 2007, after ACOG announced its new policy on universal access to prenatal testing, Stephanie Meredith began to explore what information sources existed for parents and pregnant couples who received a Down syndrome diagnosis. She found that the available options were inadequate and so decided to create her own. Meredith was well suited for the task—she had trained in technical writing and rhetoric, and her son Andy has Down syndrome. From her contacts in Down syndrome communities, Meredith knew that unhelpful, negative, and painful diagnostic experiences remained common among families. Fellow parents continued to describe pessimistic clinicians providing inaccurate and narrowly pathological characterizations of Down syndrome. These were "flashbulb" moments, which parents remembered vividly for years. Advocates, and some clinicians, knew that these initial diagnostic encounters could shape parents' perceptions of their child and the nature of their disabilities for years to come.

Mindful of these experiences and realities, Meredith wanted to create a short and digestible but comprehensive booklet that would provide biomedical information, as well as psychosocial knowledge about individuals and families with Down syndrome—all based on peer-reviewed research. Meredith developed relationships with clinicians to review the booklet and drew from work by genetic counselor Kathryn Sheets to guide her in presenting all needed perspectives. She also wanted to include photos of children with Down syndrome who were engaged in everyday activities, which were taken by photographers with the condition.[54]

A few years earlier, Democratic Senator Edward Kennedy and Republican Senator Sam Brownback had introduced the "Prenatally and Postnatally Diagnosed Conditions Awareness Act" in the US Congress. Though it had languished initially, ACOG's policy change on prenatal diagnosis created bipartisan interest. Prominent family advocates, including Will and Skotko, also played a major role in the bill's eventual passage in 2008. The Act required that women who received a new diagnosis of Down syndrome or some other prenatally or postnatally diagnosed condition be given up-to-date, evidence-based, written information about the range of physical, developmental, educational, and psychosocial outcomes for people diagnosed with the condition by a health care provider, as well as contact information for community services, including family support groups.[55] Importantly, the law created an established channel for distributing written information on disabilities, by requiring clinicians to do so immediately after diagnosis.

Following passage, the Joseph P. Kennedy Jr. Foundation specifically provided funding to produce written materials on Down syndrome. The Kennedy Foundation had been a significant contributor to disability research and support for 50 years (chapter 2). To begin, the Foundation surveyed what resources already existed—in search of a starting point. Skotko and Will found Meredith's booklet, *Understanding a Down Syndrome Diagnosis*, to be the best option. From here, the Down Syndrome Consensus Group, which had its origins in Edwards's consensus conference, began the intensive and contentious process of revising the booklet to make it acceptable to clinical professionals and major Down syndrome advocacy groups.[56]

The group debated every word, comma, and picture, but according to Skotko, "The big testing point was abortion. . . . [Must] the materials reference the fact that abortion was a legal option, or not?" Clinicians in the Consensus Group believed that their colleagues would only accept and distribute the materials if they did not perceive the booklet as "parent propaganda." Further, obstetricians refused to offer their endorsement if abortion was not identified as a legal option, along with pregnancy continuation and adoption. At the same time, some NDSS and NDSC leaders had strong pro-life views and resisted mentioning selective abortion for Down syndrome. Skotko noted that, because AGOC's approval was necessary for success, the Down syndrome advocacy groups "very begrudgingly" accepted the inclusion of abortion.[57]

The collectively approved revision of Meredith's *Understanding a Down Syndrome Diagnosis* (hereafter called the "Lettercase booklet," after the non-profit organization that later published and distributed it) was first distributed in 2011. It featured endorsements by the two major national Down syndrome advocacy groups, as well as ACOG, NSGC, and ACMG. Unfortunately, the consensus was tenuous and quickly dissolved. NDSC's and NDSS's misgivings about their initial compromise on abortion were amplified in late 2011 by the clinical launch of noninvasive prenatal screening. These techniques collected fetal DNA from the maternal blood to detect the presence of extra chromosomes, including trisomy 21—the cause of Down syndrome. Noninvasive screening revolutionized the prenatal testing landscape by offering high-sensitivity results with no risk of miscarriage. For a pregnant woman, the test seemed like just another blood draw, making it quite distinct from invasive approaches like amniocentesis.[58] Down syndrome advocates were concerned that noninvasive screening would greatly expand the number of women undergoing prenatal testing for Down syndrome, perhaps without even realizing that they were doing so, and then choosing abortion based on the results.

In late 2012, NDSC and NDSS retracted their endorsement of the Lettercase booklet, and Skotko was suddenly removed from the NDSS board of directors. Madeline Will also left NDSS. Both national Down syndrome societies removed any mention of the Lettercase booklet from their websites, and NDSC began work on its own materials. David Tolleson, the executive director of NDSC, explained: "We don't feel it's appropriate to promote the value of those with Down syndrome while at the same time also discussing the possibility of abortion. . . . Our self-advocates told us that it was not appropriate in a pamphlet coming from their advocacy organization to talk about abortion as co-equal to any other option."[59] NDSC's own booklet made no mention of abortion. It stated that women might choose prenatal testing to "gather more information about the chance for Down syndrome in their pregnancy, and / or so they can plan for the delivery of a child with Down syndrome."[60] Skotko characterized it as "filled with factual inaccuracies and unbalanced information, which has not been peer-reviewed."[61] Tolleson countered that people already knew about selective abortion, so it did not need to be mentioned.

While it is likely that some Down syndrome self-advocates in NDSC were vocally troubled by references to abortion in the Lettercase booklet, Skotko and Meredith noted that Tolleson offered no supporting evidence or self-advocate representatives to espouse this view. NDSS and NDSC were professional and family advocacy organizations and did not have self-advocates in leadership roles. Just as self-advocates were not included in Edwards's consensus conference or the Down Syndrome Consensus Group, it is likely that individuals with Down syndrome played a very limited role in NDSC's decision to abandon the Lettercase booklet.

The dissolution of consensus had wide-ranging implications for the distribution of standardized information. Meredith noted that the existence of disagreement and competing booklets further empowered prenatal testing companies. As she put it,

> It helps when we are all on the same page. The [diagnostic] labs have used this as an excuse. They say, "We are not going to disseminate your resources because we are hearing one thing from the advocacy groups and another thing from the consensus group, so we are just not going to do anything." . . . When you are trying to reach 75,000 clinicians, and you are out-funded by hundreds of millions of dollars, the only thing you have is a unified voice to possibly address it, and we don't have that either.

The landscape for standardized information provision was further complicated by state legislation. A number of US states passed their own Prenatally and Postnatally Diagnosed Conditions Awareness Acts, beginning with

Massachusetts in 2012. Other states, including Kentucky, Pennsylvania, and Ohio, also passed versions based on the Massachusetts model. Beginning in 2014, however, similar bills were introduced in Louisiana, Texas, and Indiana with an added provision—the information provider "shall not engage in discrimination based on disability or genetic variation by explicitly or implicitly presenting pregnancy termination as a neutral or acceptable option." Notably, Down syndrome advocacy groups had not introduced these bills. Rather, they came from pro-life organizations—who did not consult the disability groups and advocates that had previously been championing such acts. In the Texas legislature, competing pro-life and disability advocacy group bills were introduced in 2015.[62]

Mark Leach, a lawyer whose daughter Juliet has Down syndrome, referred to the Louisiana Down Syndrome Information Act as a "Trojan Horse" for pro-life information, which had the effect of making clinicians even more suspicious of advocates' goals. Meredith noted that the pro-information disability advocacy movement had been "co-opted for political reasons."[63] Pro-life efforts continued with the passage of laws, beginning in North Dakota, which specifically made selective abortion to prevent Down syndrome or other disabilities illegal—with criminal and professional penalties for the physicians involved. Historian David M. Perry, whose son Nico has Down syndrome, criticized the sponsors of these bills for intentionally seeking to create a "wedge" that would divide pro-life and pro-choice disability advocates.[64]

Similar Down syndrome abortion bans also passed in Ohio, Louisiana, Indiana, and Kentucky. While such laws seemed likely at the time to be overruled by courts, their presence on the books had chilling effects on how clinical professionals spoke to patients about reproductive options. At Lettercase, which was housed in Kentucky, Meredith needed to take this legislative trend into consideration when revising *Understanding A Down Syndrome Diagnosis*. She noted that "we ended up turning the pregnancy termination section into a general coping with loss section. . . . So the resources we provide include people who may have lost babies for lots of different reasons. That was also a good way to deal with political issues involving the states that passed laws specifically prohibiting termination." Instead of directly addressing abortion, the Lettercase booklet mentioned "pregnancy management options" and "reproductive decisions."[65]

Looked at from one perspective, state laws banning condition-specific selective abortion were interventions that promised to alter perceptions about the acceptable responses to a Down syndrome diagnosis. These acts were in some ways comparable to the Reagan Administration's Baby Doe Rules, which originated in pro-life circles and discouraged medical decisions that were viewed as discriminatory because they resulted in the deaths of newborn disabled children (chapter 2). The Baby Doe Rules were widely opposed by clinicians and eventually struck down by the US Supreme Court, but they still influenced parallel legislation and sent a clear societal message that certain approaches to preventing disabilities were no longer acceptable.[66] Proponents of Down syndrome abortion bans pointed to similar goals of changing social norms through new laws but did so by limiting individuals' reproductive options during pregnancy.

Importantly, though, many families who had disabled members opposed disorder-specific abortion bans because family members did not believe that the well-being of their disabled kin was a pro-life or pro-choice issue. Rachel Adams, whose son Henry has Down syndrome, argued, "These laws trivialize the often-wrenching decision to terminate a pregnancy by suggesting that women are acting out of simple prejudice. But women decide to abort after a diagnosis of Down syndrome for many reasons. Doubtless some are motivated by misunderstanding or fear. . . . But many others believe they lack the resources required for such a child to flourish." As Adams and other disability advocates pointed out, some state legislatures also passed bills that reduced existing benefits for developmental disabilities during the same session as their abortion bans. When Pennsylvania governor Tom Wolf vetoed a similar condition-specific abortion ban in 2019, he noted that he was not aware of a single disability rights group that had supported it.[67]

Facilitating Choice in a Changing Environment

New state laws in the late 2010s had a chilling effect on what genetic counselors and other clinicians felt empowered to discuss with their patients and how honest people could be with genetic counselors about their reproductive considerations and intentions. The primary purpose of genetic counseling was to describe and discuss choices. If women no longer had viable reproductive options or felt that they could not reasonably consider them, then the need for genetic counselors to help them explore their perceptions of disability was greatly diminished. Importantly, this erased a key opportunity for genetic counselors to engage families with more informative and optimistic views of disability, independent of their pregnancy outcomes.

For genetic counselors, politically induced barriers were compounded by the growing use of noninvasive screening after 2011. Historically, one of the primary justifications for prenatal genetic counseling was the risk for miscarriage associated with amniocentesis. Since noninvasive screening did not pose this risk, it seemed likely to become part of the standard of care—with no pretest counseling or any distinct consenting process.[68] Even if genetic counselors continued to provide counseling to some people *after* screening results had suggested an increased likelihood for disabilities, an important opportunity to openly discuss disability-related assumptions and concerns with *most* pregnant couples—before any testing took place—had already been missed.

Realistically, most pregnant couples probably were not all that enthusiastic about having a potentially difficult and awkward conversation with a genetic counselor concerning their perceptions and feelings about having a disabled child *before* receiving such a diagnosis took place. If the primary role and identity of genetic counselors centered around conveying biomedical information and discussing whatever patients wanted, then encouraging difficult conversations about disability could be seen as overly "directive" or even a form of biased political advocacy in the clinic (chapter 3). Genetic counselor Ellyn Farrelly noted that most patients preferred to avoid such deep conversations about disability, but she suggested,

> We need to spend more time asking, "What's important to you? What's your vision for the future? What are your hopes for your family?" And then talking through, "If a concern arises during the pregnancy, what would you like to do at that point?" "If you have a child that has some learning difference, what do you think about that? How do you feel about that?"

As Farrelly saw it, just because many patients were not comfortable with talking about disability-related considerations did not mean that genetic counselors had no professional responsibility to bring up these topics.[69]

Another genetic counselor insightfully suggested to me that a way to prepare patients for potentially difficult conversations about disability would be to place some leading questions on their intake form. It might begin by stating, "About 3 percent of babies are born with some form of disability" and then list a series of *yes* or *no* questions, with room left for elaboration. Potential questions could include: Are you concerned about your child having a disability? Do you believe that your family has the resources to cope

with disability? Would you like more information about community resources for children with disabilities? Have you had close relations with a
disabled child or adult? If so, do you feel positive about the family support
and resources that have been available for them? Could you imagine raising
a similar child yourself? If possible, would you like to know in advance that
your baby will have disabilities?

These questions would help to ease the patient into thinking about their
views and knowledge of disabilities and would give their genetic counselor
some background information as a starting point to begin a larger conversation. Patients might still be uncomfortable or resistant to discussing disability, but the mere introduction of this topic could encourage them to
reconsider some of their assumptions.

One opening for engaging with disability perspectives in a genetic counseling session could be pursued when patients ask the dreaded question,
"What would you do in my situation?" Historically, many genetic counselors
were taught to deflect or to answer that they cannot know what the patient
should do without "being in their shoes." Another potential interpretation
of this question would be that the patient is probing the genetic counselor
for a better sense of what is a socially acceptable or appropriate response
to the situation, decision, or challenge that they face. In this context, the
patient may assume that the genetic counselor has a more accurate sense of
what most people do in these circumstances, or the patient views the counselor as a gatekeeper of sorts for socially appropriate actions and broader
societal views on complex issues—like selective abortion. As potential advocates for disabled people, genetic counselors could do more to embrace this
question as a valuable educational opportunity. It can be a chance to provide
more optimistic narratives of life with a disability, which might be entirely
absent from a patient's assumptions and perspectives. There are no neutral
answers to this question, but there are responses that promote more positive, inclusive, and sociopolitical understandings of disabled people.

Conclusions

Keeping conversations open was an important ambition and achievement for disability self-advocates in their ongoing engagement with genetic
counselors. Their efforts established novel forums for dialogue and led to
greater understanding and empathy in the fraught area of prenatal diagnosis and disability rights. Self-advocates sought to enhance genetic counselors'

exposure to the lived experiences and perspectives of disabled people and their families and hoped that more genetic counselors would become disability advocates themselves—promoting more positive and accepting narratives in the prenatal setting and society more broadly. Genetic counselors will always face pressure to learn about and respond to the latest genetic technologies and testing policies. Importantly, ongoing dialogue with self-advocates about various disability communities' more general views of genetic testing and selective abortion can provide genetic counselors with a consistent, values-based framework for addressing new innovations.

As I describe in this chapter, disability self-advocates had notable success in shaping a few genetic counseling training programs and thus creating models for greater disability engagement in others. When it came to pushing for change within NSGC, however, the achievements of self-advocates and their allies in genetic counseling were more limited. NSGC's leadership remained focused on highlighting genetic counselors' professional role as patient educators and facilitators of decision-making, and their identity as biomedical experts and protectors of reproductive choice. They generally avoided sociopolitical advocacy—except when it came to defending abortion rights. Disability advocates could not convince NSGC to acknowledge that selective abortion had discriminatory impacts on disabled people, or to seriously reconsider the implications of its close relationships with abortion providers and genetic testing corporations.

After 2010, the landscape of prenatal genetic counseling began to change, as various technological and political developments preempted important discussions about disability in the prenatal context. Amid this, genetic counselors and disability advocates increasingly came to appreciate the overlapping nature of their goals and challenges. Disability self-advocates had long promoted the idea that more positive and inclusive narratives of life with disabilities would encourage fewer people to choose selective abortion. They also believed that transforming the decision to give birth to a disabled child from a family's choice into a state-enforced requirement ran counter to their own personal values and actually hurt their ambitions to make society more knowledgeable, accepting, and optimistic about the experiences of disabled individuals.

With the introduction of new pro-life legislative strategies, genetic counselors increasingly came to appreciate that—like access to abortion—the provision and discussion of clinical knowledge was also a sociopolitical issue.

As disability self-advocates had been saying all along, the explanations and conversations that genetic counselors offered in the prenatal context were not neutral and nondirective. Whether genetic counselors acknowledged it or not, disability-related discussions and decisions were highly political activities, which could be targeted by interest groups with a wide diversity of goals. Limits on what genetic counselors could openly discuss with their patients—along with technological changes that made such conversations seem less necessary—not only threatened them professionally but also impacted their central ambition of promoting widely available and fully informed reproductive choices.

Synthesis and Next Steps

Chapters 4, 5, and 6 each offer case studies of efforts by clinical professionals to dismiss or tame the sociopolitical views and advocacy of other interest groups. Clinical psychologists defended the priority and prestige of their scientific ways of knowing and approaches by resisting sociopolitical advocacy that sought to ban dehumanizing interventions, alter the orientation of classification schemes, and encourage new perspectives on the true potential of people with "severe" developmental disabilities. Meanwhile, neurodevelopmental disabilities specialists in pediatrics maintained that their narrowly biological conceptions best served patients with "chronic brain damage" and that these children were bound to fall through the cracks if they ended up in the jurisdiction of clinicians with stronger psychosocial or political orientations. Similarly, genetic counselors viewed disability self-advocates' perspectives on the sociopolitical impacts of prenatal diagnosis and selective abortion as conflicting with their professional commitment to informing and facilitating autonomous reproductive choices. In each case, clinicians saw clear professional benefits in resisting more positive, accepting, and sociopolitical narratives of disabled people, while also arguing that they were acting in the best interests of their patients by defending the legitimacy and prestige of their long-standing professional roles and approaches. Clinicians saw many advantages in maintaining the status quo.

The epilogue of this book introduces additional perspectives from disabled people who themselves trained to be clinical professionals. I examine the ongoing barriers to disabled individuals succeeding in clinical professional training programs and careers, while making the case that having more disabled clinical practitioners would help to encourage their clinical professional students, colleagues, and patients to reconsider their existing views of disabled people. Disabled clinicians are uniquely situated to combine their extensive training in biomedical knowledge and approaches with their lived experiences of disability as a social and political identity and make arguments that are difficult for others to easily dismiss.

Epilogue

The Need for Disabled Clinical Professionals

Cynthia Parker felt confident about her chances. The admissions committee had told her that they were interviewing ten people for six slots—and that some of the candidates would be wait-listed. This seemed like good odds for a highly regarded graduate program in a competitive field. At worst, Parker figured, she would end up on the waiting list. A few weeks later, she was surprised to receive a rejection letter. What had happened? Why was she not put on the waiting list? Was it her grades, or was it because she was disabled? Parker still wondered about this outcome over a decade later—long after she had graduated from another program and started her career. Just as these things usually went, she recalled, "I didn't ask why, of course, and they didn't say."

Numerous disabled people have had similar experiences in the professional world. Although this opening anecdote really happened (to someone with a different name), there is no need for me to identify in which clinical field, when, or even what form of outward disability was involved. Stories like this were very common across the postwar clinical professions—even in recent decades. Admissions committees often asked potential trainees about how they would prevent their disability status from affecting their professional judgment and objectivity. Applicants and students were blamed for a sign language interpreter's lack of biomedical knowledge. They were denied access to a necessary support—even if they offered to pay for it themselves—sometimes with the justification that "people like them did not belong in medicine."

Disabled trainees often experienced negative and unaccommodating attitudes from teachers and supervisors. They were dismissed as incapable to

practice because they could not perform traditional but completely unnecessary exercises, like placing a surgical retractor. Sometimes, graduates accepted
work as an unpaid volunteer at first, because they had to prove that they could
do the job. Several disabled clinicians left their field due to its discriminatory
culture—some after being denied jobs suited to their expertise—or because
they saw little potential for career advancement. It was not uncommon for
disabled clinicians to work for one employer for several years, but after the
employer's retirement to find that no one else was willing to hire them, despite their extensive experience. Importantly though, many disabled people
did finish their graduate programs and internships, and did find fulfilling
work, and did have long, successful careers.[1]

During the late twentieth century, landmark legislation, including Section 504 of the Rehabilitation Act and the Americans with Disabilities Act,
increased the likelihood that disabled individuals would be accepted and
supported as clinical professional trainees. Yet, like many other historically
marginalized minority groups, disabled people remain poorly represented
in the clinical professions. They also continue to face subtle and direct questions about whether they belong in clinical careers and if they can "safely"
and adequately serve patients and thrive professionally. Clinical professions
have not actively recruited disabled trainees to the same extent, if at all, as
they have worked since 1968 to include more women and racial minorities.
As self-advocates have long argued, disabled people still struggle to overcome societal and professional assumptions that they are biologically deficient and thus unqualified for certain roles.[2] In this chapter, I examine and
compare the histories and future potentials of clinical psychology, pediatrics,
and genetic counseling to adopt more positive, inclusive, and sociopolitical
views of disability and consider how disabled clinicians can and do serve as
powerful agents of change.

Barriers and Pathways to Change

My historical examination of three distinct clinical disciplines reveals
more continuities than divergences in terms of evolving understandings
and approaches to disabled people, as well as practitioners' and professional
organizations' responses to more positive, inclusive, and sociopolitical perspectives on disability. This was the case despite significant differences among
these disciplines in terms of scientific commitments and interests, field size,
degree type, relationship to medicine, and prestige in the status hierarchy of

health care and biomedicine. In general, reluctant responses to more optimistic and accepting views of life with disabilities were commonplace and long-standing. Still, noticeable advancements in the adoption of new disability narratives did take place in each field, although often slowly and unevenly. On the whole, disability perspectives in the clinical professions studied were reformed but not revolutionized.

The evolution of postwar clinical approaches to disability was much more in line with "biopsychosocial model" alternatives to the "medical model" than the transformative viewpoints of newer "social model" and "diversity model" perspectives (introduction). Since the 1970s, biopsychosocial reformers in the clinical professions have sought to increase consideration of the contributions of psychological and socioenvironmental factors to medical problems—although while still privileging biological explanations and individual-level interventions. Biopsychosocial proponents often overlooked the harms of medicalization for disabled people and their communities, as well as the impacts of clinicians' paternalistic attitudes toward disability self-advocacy. These clinicians generally did not see a role for themselves in sociopolitical disability advocacy beyond the clinic, or outside of their biomedical expertise.[3]

Meanwhile, social model proponents, many of who were self-advocates, reframed disability as being caused by societal stigma and oppression. They called for and led political advocacy efforts to bring about changes in governmental, professional, and institutional policies and perspectives. The diversity model (chapter 1) further added that disabled people should celebrate their unique traits and experiences and suggested that clinicians could help their patients recognize and embrace a disability identity. Although some clinical professionals—and in particular disabled practitioners—championed or adopted these more revolutionary perspectives, most remained resistant to, unresponsive to, or unaware of their potential impacts.[4]

Scholars have frequently and productively contrasted "social model" versus "medical model" conceptions of disability. In doing so, however, they have often characterized the latter in ahistorical and one-dimensional ways. From its origins in the 1950s, the medical model was primarily mobilized to critique medical assumptions and approaches and to call for reform or revolution. Importantly, postwar clinicians rarely defended the medical model or pointed it as an intentional approach to training and practice.[5] My historical analysis in this book pushes beyond the assumption that clinical professionals rejected new views of disability simply due to their allegiance to the "medical model." Instead, I examine clinicians' reluctant responses to more positive, inclusive, and sociopolitical perspectives on disabled people—which scholars have long attributed to the medical model—by taking account of other complex and evolving motivations, which were informed by concerns about professional role, identity, and prestige. I argue that, to adequately understand and address barriers to more revolutionary change in medicine and society, scholars must do more to consider the specific sources and manifestations of professional opposition to alternative "social" and "diversity" model narratives of disability.

In this book, I highlight a number of important avenues and barriers to greater change in the postwar clinical professions. First and foremost, disability self-advocates and family advocates had a powerful role in introducing and promoting more positive and inclusive perspectives on disabled people and lives among clinical professionals. It is difficult to imagine that similar progress toward more optimistic, accepting, and sociopolitical views of disability would have taken place without the persistent efforts of these advocates. Postwar legislative advances also had some impact on policies and approaches. Notably, clinical professional organizations often lagged in their awareness and implementation of laws like the Education for All Handicapped Children Act (PL 94-142) and the Americans with Disabilities Act. Clinicians jumped into action much more quickly when they felt threatened— as pediatricians did by the Baby Doe Rules and genetic counselors did by anti-abortion politics. In general, new laws subtly reshaped the clinical professions in limited but still important ways. By the 1980s, allowing newborn disabled children to die unnecessarily had become no longer acceptable, and professional associations had begun to acknowledge that disabled trainees and clinicians had the legal right to some accommodations.

Amid these changes, clinicians viewed new perspectives on disability as incongruous or imperiling to their identity, role, and prestige. To help maintain and bolster these important professional considerations, each discipline highlighted its expert status and mastery of abstract scientific knowledge, theory, and methodologies.[6] More optimistic and inclusive disability narratives often came in conflict with or outright challenged the assumptions and products of these privileged biomedical ways of knowing—especially when it came to defining causes, characterizing "severity," and recommending or assessing interventions. Clinicians also focused on individual-level engagement, advocacy, and treatments for disabled people, while rarely pursuing activities that brought them outside of the clinic or their biomedical expertise. Extra-clinical roles and political advocacy were rarely emphasized during training, were unlikely to lead to career advancement, and could be seen as biased or compromising to professional objectivity.

Interpretations of severity played a consistently central role in how clinical professionals engaged with disability and resisted calls for reform or revolutionary change. The label of "severe" disabilities was used by clinicians to delineate specialty areas and jurisdictions, to identify disabled individuals as biologically deficient and unlikely to be cared for or helped by other clinicians, to warrant extreme interventions while dismissing the viability of others, and to justify the ongoing use of "preventive" interventions involving selective abortion or intentional starvation. Some bioethicists contributed to the prevalence and apparent practicality of thinking about disabilities in terms of severity by attempting to establish seemingly objective and ethical standards for "line drawing" between differing forms of disability. Disability self-advocates and family advocates, some of who were bioethicists themselves, played an important role in critiquing these efforts to delineate "severe" disabilities, while noting the inaccuracies, subjectivity, and ableism inherent in these clinical and bioethical judgments.[7] Throughout this book, I have pointed to pronouncements about the severity of disabilities as a significant barrier to more optimistic, inclusive, and sociopolitical disability perspectives, as well as a common means for justifying oppressive, painful, dehumanizing, nihilistic, and deadly policies and interventions.

Comparing Clinical Disciplines

Engagement with novel ways of viewing and interpreting disability was influenced by the unique characteristics of each discipline studied in this book. While all three fields were strongly invested and dependent on their scientific identities, particular interests within each varied. Genetic counseling's close ties to genetic testing forced the field to constantly keep up with new innovations, products, and policies—most of which encouraged more reductive thinking about disabilities, especially in the prenatal setting. At the same time, some genetic counselors and medical geneticists were highly invested in specific genetic conditions and formed close relationships with affected families while engaging in sociopolitical advocacy beyond the clinic. Pediatricians' focus on the science of child development led to more psychosocially and environmentally based views of certain disabilities but also to divisive competition over professional recognition and jurisdiction. Within clinical psychology, scientific commitments and investments varied widely, from strict behaviorist to highly sociopolitical orientations.

The large size and heterogeneity of the psychology discipline stands out as a significant factor in clinical psychologists' varying views and approaches to disability. Larger disciplines have the potential to more comfortably accommodate a wider range of epistemologies and practices, although in clinical psychology, some of these were certainly more prestigious than others. Compared to clinical psychology, postwar pediatrics and genetic counseling were more intellectually homogeneous fields, and the latter was much smaller. Simply put, there were fewer ways to become, or be, a postwar pediatrician or genetic counselor than what the discipline of psychology offered its trainees and clinicians. These trends began with limited epistemic and experiential diversity in training programs—and then fewer pathways to pursue, identities to adopt, and literatures to contribute to for pediatricians and especially genetic counselors. Pediatricians could choose a subspecialty, but most of these were narrowly oriented around organ systems and laboratory methods. In psychology, more professional divisions and niches were available to nurture diverse viewpoints—creating numerous opportunities to push the envelope on disability.

As a smaller, more homogeneous field, late twentieth-century genetic counseling probably had the best potential for a quick and relatively universal transformation toward greater investment in positive, accepting, and sociopolitical disability advocacy. The National Society of Genetic Counselors chose not to move in this direction. Rather, the field's leaders invested in highlighting a professional role and identity in educating patients and facilitating autonomous reproductive decisions. Unlike in the larger fields of pediatrics and clinical psychology, genetic counselors did not have alternative national-level professional organizations that they could turn to in seeking to pursue more optimistic disability perspectives and inclusive political aims.

Terminal degree type and relative position in the hierarchy of clinical professions were also important factors in shaping how clinical professionals did, or could, embrace new disability narratives. Clinical psychologists, with their PhD (and later PsyD, an applied clinical degree) credentialing, had the most independence to pursue new intellectual approaches and professional ambitions. Throughout the postwar period, clinical psychology fostered a professional identity and training mechanisms that were separate from medicine. At the same time, doctoral programs in postwar psychology tended to have a strong empirical research emphasis, most often privileging quantitative, laboratory-based, and controlled experimental approaches—all of which focused on individuals. Psychological research frequently presumed or reinforced pessimistic views of disability and assigned lesser value to studies incorporating disability community viewpoints or empowerment.

Master's trained genetic counselors—many of who were employed or supervised by physicians, medical institutions, or in more recent decades by genetic testing companies—were more dependent than psychologists on their identity as health care professionals. This led to a general hesitancy to invest in areas like psychosocial counseling and sociopolitical disability advocacy, which did not appear to be valued by other biomedical professionals and heath care organizations. That said, by the mid-1990s, the genetic counseling field had gained significant independence over its professional training and ambitions—after the field developed its own certification board and code of ethics. This put genetic counselors in a much stronger and autonomous position to make significant changes to their discipline's views, engagement, and approaches to disabled people, perhaps without altering the field's primary identity, role, and prestige from the vantage point of other more powerful and preeminent clinical disciplines.

Among the three disciplines I examine in this book, postwar pediatrics was the most prominent and, going forward, is probably in the best position to take the lead in introducing and promoting new disability narratives in the clinic, among patients, and in society. However, as a specialty within the American medical establishment, pediatrics may also have the most to lose from significant change. Campaigns to embrace more revolutionary disability perspectives, in place of predominant biomedical views that highlight individual pathologies and impairments, would likely face strong internal pushback in pediatrics and resistance from other specialties. The subspecialty structure of pediatrics does provide opportunities to make major changes in some training, research, and practice areas—perhaps without significantly altering the others, at first. Over time, broader impacts on pediatrics and general medical education may be possible.

What will evolution toward more positive, inclusive, and sociopolitical perspectives on disability look like in the future? The answers are likely to vary by discipline. More universal change may be necessary in smaller, more homogeneous fields like genetic counseling, but along the way, outlier programs like those at Brandeis University and Johns Hopkins / National Institutes of Health may help to model new pathways. Progress in larger disciplines, like psychology, is likely to be more sporadic and extreme. Such trends will benefit disabled people who receive care and attention from more optimistic and accepting subfields and practitioners. Meanwhile, many other individuals may be harmed if similarly transformative countervailing trends take place in other subdisciplinary areas, such as behavioral or experimental psychology.

Transitions in pediatrics will likely begin at the level of subspecialties and fellowship programs. Investments to help Developmental and Behavioral Pediatrics and other more community-oriented subspecialities, like adolescent medicine,[8] grow and expand their reach would certainly help. Increased emphasis on psychosocial and sociopolitical views of disability in fellowship training curricula will also be important, especially in relation to the wide range of developmental disabilities. Because pediatric subspecialities and postgraduate fellowship programs play a central role in shaping future trainees, investments at this level could quickly trickle down to improved training and clinical rotation experiences in more positive, inclusive, and sociopolitically oriented disability services for pediatrics residents and medical students.

The Impacts of Disabled Clinical Professionals

Considerations of professional identity, role, and prestige will likely remain, in the decades ahead, major barriers to new more positive, inclusive, and sociopolitical views of disability. While there are many pathways and opportunities available to hasten change, one of the most promising involves recruiting, accepting, and fully supporting more disabled individuals into clinical professional training programs and careers. Disabled clinicians are in a unique position to combine their biomedical expertise with their lived experiences of disability as a social and political issue and identity. They are also powerfully situated to help challenge the resistance of their colleagues, students, and patients to more optimistic disability narratives.

In making this argument, I build on disability scholars and self-advocates' previous assertions about the value and importance of welcoming and supporting more disabled people into the clinical professions.[9] As Tom Shakespeare, Lisa Iezzoni, and Nora Groce have argued, "Learning alongside a student who is a wheelchair user or has restricted growth or is deaf can challenge negative assumptions directly. . . . [It] is comparable to when physician training programs were expanded to include more women."[10] In general, greater diversity in gender, race, and other social identities contribute positively to enhancing professional cultures, perspectives, and patient care.[11] In particular, because clinicians play such a central role in defining societal conceptions and approaches to disability, the multifaceted and experientially informed views that disabled clinical professionals bring to their field can be uniquely significant and influential.

Disabled clinicians offer valuable lived and practical knowledge, as well as empathetic care and support to their disabled coworkers, trainees, and patients. They may also choose to take on active roles in promoting more positive, inclusive, and sociopolitically oriented views of disability in various biomedical contexts.[12] Additionally, disabled clinical professionals can powerfully challenge the preexisting and sometimes unrecognized presumptions of their colleagues, students, and patients about what a capable, effective, and knowledgeable clinician looks like. Their achievements demonstrate what is possible for disabled children's futures, especially if more optimistic narratives of disability are widely adopted and more inclusive policies implemented. The combination of disability worldviews and established biomedical expertise that disabled clinicians possess may facilitate more productive collaboration and encourage greater tolerance for multiple ways of knowing among their colleagues, students, academic institutions, and disciplines. Importantly, this may help to diminish the influence of competing professional considerations and concerns in clinical and research approaches.

Disabled individuals are already important proponents and agents of change in the clinical professions. Growing numbers of disabled clinical professionals will also be a key measure of broader transformations in clinical disciplines during the decades ahead. Enhanced efforts to recruit and retain disabled people in clinical professional careers will reflect increased acceptance and investment in more optimistic and inclusive disability narratives. As the roles and identities of many clinical professions become more disability-tolerant and celebratory, more disabled people may be drawn to pursue clinical careers—having seen that clinicians can provide diverse and positive support to disability communities and play an important role in countering oppressive, reductive, and pessimistic narratives about life with disabilities.

It would be misleading to suggest that greater acceptance and successes for disabled people in clinical professional careers alone would represent a panacea—addressing all ableism in medicine. Indeed, disabled clinicians face many of the same professional considerations and pressures as their colleagues. Rather, in this book, I describe the important and influential roles of disabled individuals and their family members in introducing and promoting new views of disability to clinical professionals. These *disability dialogues* had the greatest impacts when clinicians viewed disabled people and their families as more than patients in need of biomedical expertise and individual-level solutions. Such conversations also had the most meaningful effects when their goals were not narrowly defined as establishing scientific validity, winning an ethical debate, or reaching consensus but rather as giving voice to a wide range of personal and clinical experiences, perspectives, and potentials. Importantly, pathways that led in the direction of more transformative changes began when clinicians engaged with the knowledge and experiences of disabled individuals and communities as being equally valuable and potentially amenable and complementary to their own well-established conceptions of what it means to live with disabilities.

Notes

Introduction

1. Kinder, John M., *Paying with Their Bodies: American War and the Problem of the Disabled Veteran* (Chicago: University of Chicago Press, 2015); Linker, Beth, *War's Waste: Rehabilitation in World War I America* (Chicago: University of Chicago Press, 2011).

2. Herman, Ellen, *The Romance of American Psychology: Political Culture in the Age of Experts* (Berkeley: University of California Press, 1995); Capshew, James H., *Psychologists on the March: Science, Practice, and Professional Identity in America, 1929–1969* (Cambridge: Cambridge University Press, 1999); Tomes, Nancy, "The Development of Clinical Psychology, Social Work, and Psychiatric Nursing: 1900–1980s," in *History of Psychiatry and Medical Psychology*, ed. Edwin Wallace IV and John Gach, 657–82 (New York: Springer, 2008).

3. Brockley, Janice, "Rearing the Child Who Never Grew: Ideologies of Parenting and Intellectual Disability in American History," in *Mental Retardation in American: A Historical Reader*, ed. James W. Trent Jr. and Steven Noll, 130–64 (New York: New York University Press, 2004); Carey, Allison C., *On the Margins of Citizenship: Intellectual Disability and Civil Rights in Twentieth-Century America* (Philadelphia: Temple University Press, 2009).

4. Stern, Alexandra Minna, *Telling Genes: The Story of Genetic Counseling in America* (Baltimore: Johns Hopkins University Press, 2012).

5. Hahn, Harlan, "The Politics of Physical Differences: Disability and Discrimination," *Journal of Social Issues* 44, no. 1 (1988): 39–47; Schweik, Susan M., *The Ugly Laws: Disability in Public* (New York: New York University Press, 2009).

6. Wolfensberger, Wolf, "Diagnosis Diagnosed," *Journal of Mental Subnormality* 11, no. 21 (1965): 62–70; Starr, Paul, *The Social Transformation of American Medicine* (New York: Basic Books, 1982).

7. Noll, Steven, and James W. Trent, *Mental Retardation in America: A Historical Reader* (New York: New York University Press, 2004); Nielsen, Kim E., *A Disability History of the United States* (Boston: Beacon Press, 2012); Hogan, Andrew J., "Medical Eponyms: Patient Advocates, Professional Interests, and the Persistence of Honorary Naming," *Social History of Medicine* 29, no. 3 (2016): 534–56; Hogan, Andrew J., "The 'Two Cultures' in Clinical Psychology: Constructing Disciplinary Divides in the Management of Mental Retardation," *Isis* 109, no. 4 (2018): 695–719.

8. For more on this in recent scholarship: Andrews, Erin E., *Disability as Diversity: Developing Cultural Competence* (New York: Oxford University Press, 2020); Virdi, Jaipreet, *Hearing Happiness: Deafness Cures in History* (Chicago: University of Chicago Press, 2020).

9. Hahn, Harlan, "Toward a Politics of Disability: Definitions, Disciplines, and Policies," *Social Science Journal* 22, no. 4 (1985): 87–105; Carey, *On the Margins of Citizenship*; Fleischer, Doris, and Frieda Zames, *The Disability Rights Movement: From Charity to Confirmation*, 2nd ed. (Philadelphia: Temple University Press, 2011).

10. Zola, Irving Kenneth, *Missing Pieces: A Chronicle of Living with a Disability* (Philadelphia: Temple University Press, 1982); Olkin, Ruth, *What Psychotherapists Should Know About Disability* (New York: Guilford Press, 1999); Wendell, Susan, *The Rejected Body: Feminist Philosophical Reflections on Disability* (New York: Routledge, 1996); Andrews, *Disability as Diversity*; Virdi, *Hearing Happiness*.

11. Epstein, Steven, *Impure Science: AIDS, Activism, and the Politics of Knowledge* (Berkeley: University of California Press, 1996); Bix, Amy Sue, "Diseases Chasing Money and Power: Breast Cancer and AIDS Activism Challenging Authority," *Journal of Policy History* 9, no. 1 (1997): 5–32; Lerner, Barron H., *The Breast Cancer Wars: Hope, Fear, and the Pursuit of a Cure in Twentieth-Century America* (Oxford: Oxford University Press, 2001); Nelson, Jennifer, *More Than Medicine: A History of the Feminist Women's Health Movement* (New York: New York University Press, 2015).

12. Longmore, Paul K., and Lauri Umansky, *The New Disability History: American Perspectives* (New York: New York University Press, 2001); Washington, Harriet A., *Medical Apartheid: The Dark History of Medical Experimentation on Black Americans from Colonial Times to the Present* (New York: Doubleday, 2006); Morning, Ann, *The Nature of Race: How Scientists Think and Teach About Human Difference* (Berkeley: University of California Press, 2011); Nelson, Alondra, *Body and Soul: The Black Panther Party and the Fight against Medical Discrimination* (Minneapolis: University of Minnesota Press, 2011).

13. Brown, Theodore M., "Minority Students and the Political Environment: A Historical Perspective," in *Minorities in Science: The Challenge for Change in Biomedicine*, ed. Vijaya L. Melnick and Franklin D. Hamilton, 41–52 (New York: Plenum Press, 1977); Odegaard, Charles E., *Minorities in Medicine: From Receptive Passivity to Positive Action, 1966–76* (New York: Josiah Macy Jr. Foundation, 1977); Rossiter, Margaret W., *Women Scientists in America: Before Affirmative Action, 1940–1972* (Baltimore: Johns Hopkins University Press, 1995); Kucklick, Henrika, and Robert E. Kohler, eds., *Science in the Field*, Osiris, vol. 11 (Chicago: University of Chicago Press, 1996); Nelson, *Body and Soul*; National Center for Science and Engineering Statistics, *Women, Minorities, and Persons with Disabilities in Science and Engineering* (Alexandria, VA: National Science Foundation, 2021).

14. Noll and Trent, *Mental Retardation in America*; Nielsen, *Disability History of the United States*; Carey, *On the Margins of Citizenship*; Shapiro, Joseph P., *No Pity: People with Disabilities Forging a New Civil Rights Movement* (New York: Three Rivers Press, 1993); Pelka, Fred, *What We Have Done: An Oral History of the Disability Rights Movement* (Amherst, MA: University of Massachusetts Press, 2012).

15. Longmore and Umansky, *New Disability History*, 7; Linker, Beth, "On the Borderland of Medical and Disability History: A Survey of the Fields," *Bulletin of the History of Medicine* 87, no. 4 (2013): 499–535.

16. Wright, David, *Downs: The History of a Disability* (New York: Oxford University Press, 2011); Stern, *Telling Genes*.

17. Galer, Dustin, *Working Towards Equity: Disability Rights Activism and Employment in Late Twentieth-Century Canada* (Toronto, ON: University of Toronto Press, 2018); Schmidt, Marion, *Eradicating Deafness? Genetics, Pathology, and Diversity in Twentieth-Century America* (Manchester, UK: Manchester University Press, 2020).

18. Hahn, "Politics of Physical Differences."

19. Abbott, Andrew, *The System of Professions: An Essay on the Division of Expert Labor* (Chicago: University of Chicago Press, 1988), 87–90.

20. Gettings, Robert M., *Forging a Federal-State Partnership: A History of Federal Developmental Disabilities Policy* (Washington, DC: American Association on Intellectual and Developmental Disabilities, 2011).

21. Jones, Kathleen W., "Education for Children with Mental Retardation: Parent Activism, Public Policy, and Family Ideology in the 1950s," in *Mental Retardation in America: A Historical Reader*, ed. Steven Noll and James W. Trent Jr., 322–50. (New York: New York University Press, 2004); Carey, *On the Margins of Citizenship*.

22. Castles, Katherine, "'Nice Average Americans': Postwar Parents' Groups and the Defense of the Normal Family," in *Mental Retardation in America: A Historical Reader*, ed. Steven Noll and James W. Trent Jr., 351–70 (New York: New York University Press, 2004), 365.

23. Mechanic, David, and David A Rochefort, "Deinstitutionalization: An Appraisal of Reform," *Annual Review of Sociology* 16 (1990): 301–27; Trent Jr., James W., *Inventing the Feeble Mind: A History of Mental Retardation in the United States* (Berkeley: University of California Press, 1994).

24. Blatt, Burton, and Fred Kaplan, *Christmas in Purgatory: A Photographic Essay on Mental Retardation* (Boston: Allyn and Bacon, 1966); Nehring, Wendy M., "Formal Health-care at the Community Level: The Child Development Clinics of the 1950s and 1960s," in *Mental Retardation in America: A Historical Reader*, ed. Steven Noll and James W. Trent Jr., 371–83 (New York: New York University Press, 2004); Rothman, David J., and Sheila M. Rothman, "The Litigator as Reformer," in *Mental Retardation in America: A Historical Reader*, ed. Steven Noll and James W. Trent Jr., 445–65 (New York: New York University Press, 2004).

25. Wolfensberger, Wolf, and Frank J. Menolascino, "Reflections on Recent Mental Retardation Developments in Nebraska: I. A New Plan, II. Implementation to Date," *Mental Retardation* 8, no. 6 (1970): 20–28; Eyal, Gil, Brendan Hart, Emine Oncular, and Neta Oren, *The Autism Matrix: The Social Origins of the Autism Epidemic* (New York: Polity Press, 2010).

26. Shapiro, *No Pity*; Fleischer and Zames, *Disability Rights Movement*; Pelka, *What We Have Done*.

27. Carey, *On the Margins of Citizenship*; Nielsen, *Disability History of the United States*.

28. Hahn, "Politics of Physical Differences"; Longmore and Umansky, *New Disability History*; Saxton, Marsha, ed., *Sticks and Stones: Disabled People's Stories of Abuse, Defiance, and Resilience* (Oakland, CA: World Institute on Disability, 2009).

29. Rapp, Rayna, and Faye D. Ginsberg, "Enabling Disability: Rewriting Kinship, Reimagining Citizenship," *Public Culture* 13, no. 3 (2001): 533–58; Estreich, George, *Fables and Futures: Biotechnology, Disability, and the Stories We Tell Ourselves* (Cambridge, MA: MIT Press, 2019).

30. Union of Physically Impaired Against Segregation, *Fundamental Principles of Disability* (London: UPIAS, 1976); Zola, *Missing Pieces*; Oliver, Michael, *The Politics of Disablement* (London: Macmillan, 1990); Shakespeare, Tom, *Disability Rights and Wrongs Revisited*, 2nd ed. (New York: Routledge, 2013).

31. Epstein, *Impure Science*; Nelson, *Body and Soul*; Lerner, *Breast Cancer Wars*; Kline, Wendy, "'Please Include This in Your Book'": Readers Respond to *Our Bodies, Ourselves*," *Bulletin of the History of Medicine* 79, no. 1 (2005): 81–110; Cowan, Ruth Schwartz, *Heredity and Hope: The Case for Genetic Screening* (Cambridge, MA: Harvard University Press, 2008).

32. Fleischer and Zames, *Disability Rights Movement*; Pelka, *What We Have Done*; Nielsen, *Disability History of the United States*.

33. Davis, Lennard J., *Enabling Acts: The Hidden Story of How the Americans with Disabilities Act Gave the Largest US Minority Its Rights* (Boston: Beacon Press, 2015); Andrews, *Disability as Diversity*.

34. Wright, *Downs*; Rapp, Rayna, and Faye Ginsberg, "Screening Disabilities: Visual Fields, Public Culture, and the Atypical Mind in the Twenty-First Century," in *Civil Disabilities: Citizenship, Membership, and Belonging*, ed. Nancy J. Hirschmann and Beth Linker, 103–22 (Philadelphia: University of Pennsylvania Press, 2015).

35. Nielsen, *Disability History of the United States*, 171–72; Maroto, Michelle, and David Pettinicchio, "Twenty-Five Years after the ADA: Situating Disability in America's System of Stratification," *Disability Studies Quarterly* 35, no. 3 (2015): 1–34.

36. Meeks, Lisa M., and Nira R. Jain, *Accessibility, Inclusion, and Action in Medical Education: Lived Experiences of Learners and Physicians with Disabilities* (Washington, DC: Association of American Medical Colleges, 2018); Jain, Nira R., "Political Disclosure: Resisting Ableism in Medical Education," *Disability & Society* 35, no. 3 (2020): 389–412.

37. Bell, Christopher M., *Blackness and Disability: Critical Examination and Cultural Interventions* (Lansing: Michigan State University Press, 2011); Lukin, Josh, "Disability and Blackness," in *The Disability Studies Reader*, 4th ed., ed. Lennard J. Davis, 308–15 (New York: Routledge, 2013).

38. Bosk, Charles, *All God's Mistakes: Genetic Counseling in a Pediatric Hospital* (Chicago: University of Chicago Press, 1992); Antommaria, Armand Matheny, "'Who Should Survive? One of the Choices on Our Conscience': Mental Retardation and the History of Contemporary Bioethics," *Kennedy Institute of Ethics Journal* 16, no. 3 (2006): 205–24; Wright, *Downs*, 161–64.

39. Lippman, Abby, "The Geneticization of Health and Illness: Implications for Social Practice," *Endocrinologie* 29, nos. 1–2 (1991): 85–90; Hogan, Andrew J., *Life Histories of Genetic Disease: Patterns and Prevention in Postwar Medical Genetics* (Baltimore: Johns Hopkins University Press, 2016); Löwy, Ilana, *Imperfect Pregnancies: A History of Birth Defects and Prenatal Diagnosis* (Baltimore: Johns Hopkins University Press, 2017); Navon, Daniel, *Mobilizing Mutations: Human Genetics in the Age of the Patient* (Chicago: University of Chicago Press, 2019).

40. Parens, Erik, and Adrienne Asch, eds., *Prenatal Testing and Disability Rights* (Washington, DC: Georgetown University Press, 2000); Mills, Carol Bishop, and Elina Erzikova, "Prenatal Testing, Disability, and Termination: An Examination of Newspaper Framing," *Disability Studies Quarterly* 32, no. 3 (2012); Saxton, Marsha, "Disability Rights and Selective Abortion," in *The Disability Studies Reader*, 4th ed., ed. Lennard J. Davis, 87–99 (New York: Routledge, 2013).

41. Rothenberg, Karen H., and Elizabeth Jean Thomson, eds:, *Women and Prenatal*

Testing: Facing the Challenges of Genetic Technology (Columbus: Ohio State University Press, 1994); Rapp, Rayna, *Testing Women, Testing the Fetus: The Social Impact of Amniocentesis in America* (New York: Routledge, 1999); Williams, Claire, Priscilla Alderson, and Bobbie Farsides, "Too Many Choices? Hospital and Community Staff Reflect on the Future of Prenatal Screening," *Social Science and Medicine* 55, no. 5 (2002): 743–53; Estreich, *Fables and Futures*.

42. Shakespeare, Tom, "'Losing the Plot'? Medical and Activist Discourses of Contemporary Genetics and Disability," *Sociology of Health & Illness* 21, no. 5 (1999): 669–88; Berube, Michael, "Disability, Democracy, and the New Genetics," in *The Disability Studies Reader*, 4th ed., ed. Lennard J. Davis, 100–114 (New York: Routledge, 2013); Hubbard, Ruth, "Abortion and Disability: Who Should and Should Not Inhabit the World?," in *The Disability Studies Reader*, 4th ed., ed. Lennard J. Davis, 74–86 (New York: Routledge, 2013); Saxton, "Disability Rights and Selective Abortion."

43. Parens and Asch, *Prenatal Testing and Disability Rights*; Skotko, Brian G., Priya S. Kishnani, and George T. Capone, "Prenatal Diagnosis of Down Syndrome: How to Best Deliver the News," *American Journal of Medical Genetics Part A* 149 (2009): 2361–67.

44. Rapp and Ginsberg, "Enabling Disability," 552.

45. Parens and Asch, *Prenatal Testing and Disability Rights*; Kuhse, Helga, and Peter Singer, "Ethics and the Handicapped Newborn Infant," *Social Research* 52, no. 3 (1985): 505–42; Buchanan, Allen, Dan W. Brock, Norman Daniels, and Daniel Wikler, *From Chance to Choice: Genetics and Justice* (Cambridge: Cambridge University Press, 2000); Asch, Adrienne, "Disability, Bioethics, and Human Rights," in *Handbook of Disability Studies*, ed. Gary L. Albrecht, Katherine D. Seelman, and Michael Bury, 297–326 (Thousand Oaks, CA: Sage, 2001); Wasserman, David, "A Choice of Evils in Prenatal Testing," *Florida State University Law Review* 30, no. 1 (2002): 295–313; Amundson, Ron, and Shari Tresky, "Bioethics and Disability Rights: Conflicting Values and Perspectives," *Journal of Bioethical Inquiry* 5, no. 2 (2008): 111–23; Stark, Laura, *Behind Closed Doors: IRBs and the Making of Ethical Research* (Chicago: University of Chicago Press, 2011).

46. Moore-West, Maggie, and Debbie Heath, "The Physically Handicapped Student in Medical School: A Preliminary Study," *Journal of Medical Education* 57, no. 12 (1982): 918–21; Wainapel, Stanley F., "The Physically Disabled Physician," *JAMA* 257, no. 21 (1987): 2935–38; French, Sally, "Experiences of Disabled Health and Caring Professionals," *Sociology of Health and Illness* 10, no. 2 (1988): 170–88.

47. Steinberg, Annie G., Lisa I. Iezzoni, Alicia Conill, Margaret Stineman, "Reasonable Accommodations for Medical Faculty with Disabilities," *JAMA* 288, no. 24 (2002): 3147–54; Neal-Boylan, Leslie et al., "The Career Trajectories of Health Care Professionals Practicing with Permanent Disabilities," *Academic Medicine* 87, no. 2 (2012): 172–78; Meeks and Jain, *Accessibility, Inclusion, and Action in Medical Education*.

48. Shakespeare, Tom, Lisa I. Iezzoni, and Nora E. Groce, "Disability and the Training of Health Professionals," *Lancet* 374 (2009): 1815–16, 1816.

49. Longmore and Umanski, *New Disability History*; Kudlick, Catherine J., "Disability History: Why We Need Another 'Other,'" *American Historical Review* 108, no. 3 (2003): 763–93; Scotch, Richard K., "'Nothing About Us Without Us': Disability Rights in America," *OAH Magazine of History* 23, no. 3 (2009): 17–22; Linker, Beth, and Nancy J. Hirschmann,

ed., *Civil Disabilities: Citizenship, Membership, and Belonging* (Philadelphia: University of Pennsylvania Press, 2015).

50. Zola, Irving Kenneth, *Socio-Medical Inquiries: Recollections, Reflections, and Reconsiderations* (Philadelphia: Temple University Press, 1983); Hahn, "Toward a Politics of Disability"; Shakespeare, Tom, "The Social Model of Disability," in *The Disability Studies Reader*, 4th ed., ed. Lennard J. Davis, 214–21 (New York: Routledge, 2013); Oliver, *Politics of Disablement*.

51. Barnes, Colin, and Geof Mercer, eds., *Exploring the Divide: Illness and Disability* (Leeds, UK: Disability Press, 1996).

52. Hogan, Andrew J., "Moving Away from the 'Medical Model': The Development and Revision of the World Health Organization's Classification of Disability," *Bulletin of the History of Medicine* 93, no. 2 (2019): 241–69; Hogan, Andrew J., "Social and Medical Models of Disability and Mental Health: Evolution and Renewal," *CMAJ* 191 (2019): E16–18.

53. Engel, George L., "The Need for a New Medical Model: A Challenge for Biomedicine," *Science* 196, no. 4286 (1977): 129–36; Zola, Irving K., "Toward the Necessary Universalizing of a Disability Policy," *Milbank Quarterly* 67, Supplement 2, Pt 2 (1989): 401–28; Bickenbach, Jerome E., Somnath Chatterji, Elizabeth M. Badley, and T. B. Ustun, "Models of Disablement, Universalism and the International Classification of Impairments, Disabilities and Handicaps," *Social Science and Medicine* 48, no. 9 (1999): 1173–87.

54. Pfeiffer, David, "The Devils Are in the Details: The ICIDH2 and the Disability Movement," *Disability and Society* 15, no. 7 (2000): 1079–82; Barnes, Colin, "Extended Review," *Disability and Society* 18, no. 6 (2003): 827–33; Imrie, Rob, "Demystifying Disability: A Review of the International Classification of Functioning, Disability and Health," *Sociology of Health and Illness* 26, no. 3 (2004): 287–305.

55. Morris, Jenny, "Personal and Political: A Feminist Perspective on Researching Physical Disability," *Disability, Handicap, and Society* 7, no. 2 (1992): 157–66; Crow, Liz, "Including All of Our Lives: Renewing the Social Model of Disability," in *Exploring the Divide: Illness and Disability*, ed. Colin Barnes and Geof Mercer, 55–73 (Leeds, UK: Disability Press, 1996); Wendell, Susan, "Unhealthy Disabled: Treating Chronic Illnesses as Disabilities," *Hypatia* 16, no. 4 (2001): 17–33; Shakespeare, Tom, Jerome E. Bickenbach, David Pfeiffer, and Nicholas Watson, "Models," in *Encyclopedia of Disability*, ed. Gary L. Albrecht, 1101–6 (Thousand Oaks, CA: Sage, 2006); Shakespeare et al., , "Disability and the Training of Health Professionals."

56. Linker, "On the Borderland"; Löwy, Ilana, *Tangled Diagnoses: Prenatal Testing, Women, and Risk* (Chicago: University of Chicago Press, 2018).

57. Morris, Jenny, *Pride Against Prejudice: Transforming Attitudes to Disability* (Philadelphia: New Society, 1991); Gill, Carol J., "Four Types of Integration in Disability Identity Development," *Journal of Vocational Rehabilitation* 9, no. 1 (1997): 39–46; Olkin, Ruth, *What Psychotherapists Should Know About Disability* (New York: Guilford Press, 1999); Forber-Pratt, Anjali J., Carlyn O. Mueller, and Erin E. Andrews, "Disability Identity and Allyship in Rehabilitation Psychology: Sit, Stand, Sign, and Show Up," *Rehabilitation Psychology* 64, no. 2 (2019): 119–29; Lund, Emily M., Rebecca C. Wilbur, and Angela M. Kuemmel, "Beyond Legal Obligation: The Role and Necessity of the Supervisor-Advocate in Creating a Socially

Just, Disability-Affirmative Training Environment," *Training and Education in Professional Psychology* 14, no. 2 (2020): 92–99.

58. Landsman, Gail, "Mothers and Models of Disability," *Journal of Medical Humanities* 26, nos. 2–3 (2005): 121–39; Mauldin, Laura, *Made to Hear: Cochlear Implants and Deaf Children* (Minneapolis: University of Minnesota Press, 2016), 3–5; Mauldin, Laura, "Precarious Plasticity: Neuropolitics, Cochlear Implants, and the Redefinition of Deafness," *Science, Technology, & Human Values* 39, no. 1 (2014): 130–53, 148; Blume, Stuart, *The Artificial Ear: Cochlear Implants and the Culture of Deafness* (New Brunswick, NJ: Rutgers University Press, 2010); Mills, Mara, "Do Signals Have Politics? Inscribing Abilities in Cochlear Implants," in *The Oxford Handbook of Sound Studies*, ed. Trevor Pinch and Karin Bijsterveld, 320–46 (New York: Oxford University Press, 2012).

59. Mendoza, Fernando S. et al., "Diversity and Inclusion Training in Pediatric Departments," *Pediatrics* 135, no. 4 (2015): 707–13; Lin, Luona, Karen Stamm, and Peggy Christidis, *Demographics of the US Psychology Workforce: Findings From the 2007–16 American Community Survey* (Washington, DC: American Psychological Association, 2018); National Society of Genetic Counselors, "Professional Status Survey 2020," https://www.nsgc.org/Policy-Research-and-Publications/Professional-Status-Survey.

Chapter 1. Clinical Psychology

1. Riger to Chair of APA Ethics Committee, August 26, 1992, January–February 1993 Correspondence Folder, Disability Committee Collection (DCC) (300-302-423, Box 1), American Psychological Association Archives (APA).

2. Riger, Alice L., "Disability Issues Stance Tests Our Ethical Integrity," *APA Monitor* 23, no. 11 (1992): 4.

3. Meyerson, Lee, "Physical Disability as a Social Psychological Problem," *Journal of Social Issues* 4, no. 4 (1948): 2–10, 6.

4. Herman, Ellen, *The Romance of American Psychology: Political Culture in the Age of Experts* (Berkeley: University of California Press, 1995); Routh, Donald K., "A History of Division 12 (Clinical Psychology): Four Score Years," in *Unification through Division: Histories of the Divisions of the American Psychological Association*, vol. 2, ed. Donald A. Dewsbury, 55–82 (Washington, DC: American Psychological Association, 1997); Capshew, James H., *Psychologists on the March: Science, Practice, and Professional Identity in America, 1929–1969* (Cambridge: Cambridge University Press, 1999); Tomes, Nancy, "The Development of Clinical Psychology, Social Work, and Psychiatric Nursing: 1900–1980s," in *History of Psychiatry and Medical Psychology*, ed. Edwin Wallace IV and John Gach, 657–82. (New York: Springer, 2008); Hogan, Andrew J., "The 'Two Cultures' in Clinical Psychology: Constructing Disciplinary Divides in the Management of Mental Retardation," *Isis* 109, no. 4 (2018): 695–719.

5. Cruickshank, William M., "Rehabilitation: Toward a Broader Spectrum," *Psychological Aspects of Disability* 17, no. 3 (1970): 149–58.

6. Olkin, Rhoda, and Constance Pledger, "Can Disability Studies and Psychology Join Hands?" *American Psychologist* 58, no. 4 (2003): 296–304.

7. Danziger, Kurt, *Constructing the Subject: Historical Origins of Psychological Research* (Cambridge: Cambridge University Press, 1990), 174; Danziger, Kurt, "The Project of an

Experimental Social Psychology: Historical Perspectives," *Science in Context* 5, no. 2 (1992): 309–28, 309; Sarason, Seymour B., *Psychology Misdirected* (New York: Free Press, 1981), 15–16.

8. Asch, Adrienne, "Personal Reflections," *American Psychologist* 39, no. 5 (1984): 551–52; Riger, "Disability Issues Stance"; Olkin and Pledger, "Can Disability Studies?"; Gill, Carol J., Donald G. Kewman, and Ruth W. Brannon, "Transforming Psychological Practice and Society: Policies That Reflect the New Paradigm," *American Psychologist* 58, no. 4 (2003): 305–12; Levinson, Freda, and Simon Parritt, "Against Stereotypes: Experiences of Disabled Psychologists," in *Disability and Psychology: Critical Introductions and Reflections*, ed. Daniel Goodley and Rebecca Lawthom, 111–22 (New York: Palgrave Macmillan, 2006); Andrews, Erin E. et al. "#Saytheword: A Disability Culture Commentary on the Erasure of 'Disability,'" *Rehabilitation Psychology* 64, no. 2 (2019): 111–18.

9. Asch, "Personal Reflections"; Task Force on Psychology and the Handicapped, "Final Report," *American Psychologist* 39, no. 5 (1984): 545–50, 549; Riger to Jane Winston, October 6, 1992, January–February 1993, Correspondence Folder (DCC, APA); Yuker, Harold E., "Variables That Influence Attitudes toward Persons with Disabilities: Conclusions from the Data," *Journal of Social Behavior and Personality* 9, no. 5 (1994): 3–22.

10. Danziger, *Constructing the Subject*, 174–78; Danziger, "Project of an Experimental."

11. Barker, Roger G., Beatrice A. Wright, and Mollie R. Gonick. *Adjustment to Physical Handicap and Illness: A Survey of the Social Psychology of Physique and Disability*, 2nd ed. (New York: Social Science Research Council, 1953), v–vi; Meyerson, Lee, "The Social Psychology of Physical Disability: 1948 and 1988," *Journal of Social Issues* 44, no. 1 (1988): 173–88; Schoggen, Phil, "Roger Garlock Barker (1903–1990)," *American Psychologist* 47, no. 1 (1992): 77–78; Wurl, Sheryl Lee, "Beatrice A. Wright: A Life History" (PhD diss., University of Tennessee, 2008).

12. Meyerson, "Social Psychology of Physical Disability"; Morris, Richard J., "Lee Meyerson (1920–2002)," *American Psychologist* 58, no. 10 (2003): 812.

13. Meyerson, "Physical Disability," 6–7; Lewin, Kurt, "The Conflict between Aristotelian and Galileian Modes of Thought in Contemporary Psychology," *Journal of General Psychology* 5, no. 2 (1931): 141–77; Hollingsworth, David Keith, Walter Cal Johnson Jr., and Stephen W. Cook, "Beatrice A. Wright: Broad Lens, Sharp Focus," *Journal of Counseling and Development* 67, no. 7 (1989): 384–93, 386–87.

14. Dewsbury, Donald A., *Unification through Division: Histories of the Divisions of the American Psychological Association*, vol. 3 (Washington, DC: American Psychological Association, 1999).

15. Dingfelder, S., "Clark Honored for Desegregation Influence, Life's Work," *APA Monitor* 35, no. 8 (2004): 59.

16. Meyerson, "Social Psychology of Physical Disability," 178.

17. Kutner, Bernard, "The Social Psychology of Disability," in *Rehabilitation Psychology: Proceedings of the National Conference on the Psychological Aspects of Disability*, ed. Walter S. Neff, 143–67 (Washington, DC: American Psychological Association, 1971), 145.

18. Kutner, "Social Psychology"; Barker, Roger G., "The Social Psychology of Physical Disability," *Journal of Social Issues* 4, no. 4 (1948): 28–38; Dembo, Tamara, "Some Problems in Rehabilitation as Seen by a Lewinian," *Journal of Social Issues* 38, no. 1 (1982): 131–39;

Meyerson, "Social Psychology of Physical Disability," 176; Fine, Michelle, and Adrienne Asch, "Disability beyond Stigma: Social Interaction, Discrimination, and Activism," *Journal of Social Issues* 44, no. 1 (1988): 3–21, 17.

19. Dembo, Tamara, "Sensitivity of One Person to Another," *Rehabilitation Literature* 25, no. 8 (1964): 231–35; Harding, Sandra, *The Science Question in Feminism* (Ithaca, NY: Cornell University Press, 1986); Fine and Asch, "Disability beyond Stigma," 12.

20. Dembo, "Sensitivity of One Person to Another"; Dunn, Dana S., Dawn M. Ehde, and Stephen T. Wegener, "The Foundational Principles as Psychological Lodestars: Theoretical Inspiration and Empirical Direction in Rehabilitation Psychology," *Rehabilitation Psychology* 61, no. 1 (2016): 1–6, 2–3.

21. Dembo, Tamara, L. Diller, W. A. Gordon, G. Leviton, and R. L. Sherr, "A View of Rehabilitation Psychology," *American Psychologist* 28, no. 8 (1973): 719–22, 720–21; Dembo, "Some Problems in Rehabilitation."

22. Dembo, "Some Problems in Rehabilitation," 135; Schmidt, Marion, *Eradicating Deafness? Genetics, Pathology, and Diversity in Twentieth-Century America* (Manchester, UK: Manchester University Press, 2020); Galer, Dustin, *Working towards Equity: Disability Rights Activism and Employment in Late Twentieth-Century Canada* (Toronto: University of Toronto Press, 2018).

23. Zola, Irving Kenneth, *Missing Pieces: A Chronicle of Living with a Disability* (Philadelphia: Temple University Press, 1982); Oliver, Michael, *Social Work with Disabled People* (London: Macmillan, 1983); Hahn, Harlan, "Toward a Politics of Disability: Definitions, Disciplines, and Policies," *Social Science Journal* 22, no. 4 (1985): 87–105.

24. Asch, Adrienne, "The Experience of Disability: A Challenge for Psychology," *American Psychologist* 39, no. 5 (1984): 529–36, 533.

25. Asch, "Personal Reflections," 551–52.

26. Correspondence / Comments Disability Resource Room, 1980–1987 Folder (DCC, APA).

27. Task Force on Psychology and the Handicapped, "Final Report," 546.

28. Task Force on Psychology and the Handicapped, "Final Report," 548–49; Committee on Disabilities and Handicaps, "Orientation Packet" (1988), 6 (DCC, APA).

29. Wright, Beatrice A., *Physical Disability: A Psychosocial Approach*, 2nd ed. (Harper and Row, 1983), xi; Hollingsworth, "Beatrice A. Wright," 386.

30. Jordan (1992) quoted in Pollard, Robert Q. Jr., "Professional Psychology and Deaf People: The Emergence of a Discipline," *American Psychologist* 51, no. 4 (1996): 389–96, 392.

31. Pollard, "Professional Psychology," 393; for more on the development of the psychology of deafness in the mid-twentieth century: Schmidt, *Eradicating Deafness?*, 78–92.

32. Gill, "Family / Professional Alliance in Rehabilitation Viewed from a Minority Perspective," *American Behavioral Scientist* 28, no. 3 (1985): 424–28, 427; Dobbs, Jean, "In Search of a New Aesthetic: Carol Gill Lights the Way," *New Mobility*, October 2001.

33. Fine, Asch, "Disability beyond Stigma," 14–15; Fine, Michelle, and Adrienne Asch, eds., *Women with Disabilities: Essays in Psychology, Culture, and Politics* (Philadelphia: Temple University Press, 1988).

34. Dorothy Thomas to Jeanette O'Sullivan, August 20, 1987. Correspondence / Comments Disability Resource Room, 1980–1987 Folder (DCC, APA).

35. Riger to Ethics Committee, August 26, 1992; Jones to Riger, December 15, 1992, Committee on Disability, Correspondence January–February 1993 Folder (DCC, APA).

36. Pickren, Wade E., and Henry Tomes, "The Legacy of Kenneth B. Clark to the APA: The Board of Social and Ethical Responsibility for Psychology," *American Psychologist* 57, no. 1 (2002): 51–59.

37. Riger to Winston, October 6, 1992.

38. Riger, "Disability Issues Stance."

39. Riger, "Disability Issues Stance"; APA, "Policy Statement on Full Participation for Psychologists with Disabilities," February 1997, http://citeseerx.ist.psu.edu/viewdoc /download?doi=10.1.1.651.804&rep=rep1&type=pdf.

40. Daughtry, Donald, Jennifer Gibson, and Arnold Abels, "Mentoring Students and Professionals with Disabilities," *Professional Psychology: Research and Practice* 40, no. 2 (2009): 201–205; Khubchandani, Anju, "Message from the Director of the Office on Disability Issues in Psychology," *APA Spotlight on Disability Newsletter*, August 2016.

41. Gill, Carol J., "Four Types of Integration in Disability Identity Development," *Journal of Vocational Rehabilitation* 9, no. 1 (1997): 39–46, 46.

42. Herman, *Romance of American Psychology*, 271.

43. Olkin, Rhoda, *What Psychotherapists Should Know about Disability* (New York: Guilford Press, 1999), viii–x.

44. Olkin, *What Psychotherapists Should Know*, 308.

45. Gill et al., "Transforming Psychological Practice, 306.

46. Olkin and Pledger, "Can Disability Studies?"

47. Gill et al., "Transforming Psychological Practice," 310.

48. Gill et al., "Transforming Psychological Practice," 310; APA, *Ethical Principles of Psychologists and Code of Conduct* (Washington, DC: American Psychological Association, 2002); Olkin and Pledger, "Can Disability Studies?"

49. Bogart, Kathleen R., and Dana S. Dunn, "Ableism Special Issue Introduction," *Journal of Social Issues* 75, no. 3 (2019): 650–54, 650.

50. Andrews, Erin E., *Disability as Diversity: Developing Cultural Competence* (New York: Oxford University Press, 2019), xv.

51. Lund, Emily M., Erin E. Andrews, and Judith M. Holt, "How We Treat Our Own: The Experiences and Characteristics of Psychology Trainees with Disabilities," *Rehabilitation Psychology* 59, no. 4 (2014): 367–75; Andrews, Erin E., and Emily M. Lund, "Disability in Psychology Training: Where Are We?," *Training and Education in Professional Psychology* 9, no. 3 (2015): 210–16; Michalski, Daniel, and Jessica Kohout, APA Center for Workforce Studies Doctoral Internship Module (2009), Table 5: Internship Obtained through APPIC by Demographic Characteristics, https://www.apa.org/workforce/publications/08-hsp /doctoral-internship/table-5.pdf.

52. Andrews and Lund, "Disability in Psychology Training," 215.

53. Crow, Liz, "Including All of Our Lives: Renewing the Social Model of Disability," in *Exploring the Divide: Illness and Disability*, ed. Colin Barnes, and Geof Mercer, 55–73 (Leeds, UK: Disability Press, 1996); Wendell, Susan, *The Rejected Body: Feminist Philosophical Reflections on Disability* (New York: Routledge, 1996); Forber-Pratt, Anjali J., Carlyn O. Mueller,

and Erin E. Andrews. "Disability Identity and Allyship in Rehabilitation Psychology: Sit, Stand, Sign, and Show Up," *Rehabilitation Psychology* 64, no. 2 (2019): 119–29, 120.

54. Forber-Pratt et al., "Disability Identity and Allyship," 119; Gill, "Four Types of Integration."

55. Forber-Pratt et al., "Disability Identity and Allyship," 124.

56. Olkin and Pledger, "Can Disability Studies?," 297.

57. Olkin and Pledger, "Can Disability Studies?," 296.

58. Cruickshank, "Rehabilitation: Toward a Broader Spectrum"; Krueger, David W. *Rehabilitation Psychology: A Comprehensive Textbook* (Rockland, MD: Aspen, 1984); Elliott, Timothy R., and Sandy E. Gramling, "Psychologists and Rehabilitation: New Roles and Old Training Models," *American Psychologist* 45, no. 6 (1990): 762–65; Frank, Robert G., and Timothy R. Elliott, eds., *Handbook of Rehabilitation Psychology* (Washington, DC: American Psychological Association, 2000); Kennedy, Paul, ed., *Oxford Handbook of Rehabilitation Psychology* (New York: Oxford University Press, 2012).

59. Wright, Beatrice A., "Spread in Adjustment to Disability," *Bulletin of the Menninger Clinic* 28, no. 4 (1964): 198–208; Kuhse, Helga, and Peter Singer, "Ethics and the Handicapped Newborn Infant," *Social Research* 52, no. 3 (1985): 505–42; Parens, Erik, and Adrienne Asch, eds., *Prenatal Testing and Disability Rights* (Washington, DC: Georgetown University Press, 2000); Buchanan, Allen, Dan W. Brock, Norman Daniels, and Daniel Wikler, *From Chance to Choice: Genetics and Justice* (Cambridge: Cambridge University Press, 2000); Amundson, Ron, and Shari Tresky, "Bioethics and Disability Rights: Conflicting Values and Perspectives," *Journal of Bioethical Inquiry* 5, no. 2 (2008): 111–23.

60. Erin Andrews, interview with author, December 8, 2020; Disabled Parenting Project: https://disabledparenting.com/.

61. Wolfensberger, Wolf, "A Contribution to the History of Normalization with a Primary Emphasis on the Establishment of Normalization in North America between 1967–1975," in *A Quarter-Century of Normalization and Social Role Valorization: Evolution and Impact*, ed. Robert J. Flynn and Raymond A. LeMay, 51–108 (Ottawa, ON: University of Ottawa Press, 1999), 58.

62. Wolfensberger, Wolf, "The Fiftieth Anniversary of What Appears to Be the World's First Doctoral Degree Program in Mental Retardation: Some Reminiscences of an Early Graduate," *Intellectual and Developmental Disabilities* 46, no. 1 (2008): 64–79.

63. Wolfensberger, "Fiftieth Anniversary of What Appears," 67.

64. Garfinkel, Harold, "Conditions of Successful Degradation Ceremonies," *American Journal of Sociology* 61, no. 5 (1956): 420–24; Goffman, Erving, *Asylums: Essays on the Social Situation of Mental Patients and Other Inmates* (Garden City, NY: Anchor Books, 1961); Goffman, Erving, *Stigma: Notes on the Management of Spoiled Identity* (New York: Simon & Schuster, 1963); Szasz, Thomas S., *The Myth of Mental Illness: Foundations of a Theory of Personal Conduct* (New York: Harper, 1961); Laing, R. D., and Aaron Esterson, *Sanity, Madness, and the Family* (London: Tavistock, 1964).

65. Wolfensberger, Wolf, and Frank J. Menolascino, "Reflections on Recent Mental Retardation Developments in Nebraska: I. A New Plan, II. Implementation to Date," *Mental Retardation* 8, no. 6 (1970): 20–28; Kugel, Robert B., and Wolf Wolfensberger,

Changing Patterns in Residential Services for the Mentally Retarded (Washington, DC: Presidents Committee on Mental Retardation, 1969).

66. Wolfensberger, Wolf, "The Principle of Normalization and Its Implications to Psychiatric Services," *American Journal of Psychiatry* 127, no. 3 (1970): 291–97, 292.

67. "Is Basket Weaving Harmful?," *Time*, October 12, 1970, 57.

68. Hogan, "'Two Cultures' in Clinical Psychology," 709–12.

69. Menolascino, Frank J., and Wolf Wolfensberger, "Evocation of Career Choices in Retardation: A Summer Work Experience and Training Program," *Mental Retardation* 5, no. 2 (1967): 37–39; Ronny Vink to Wolf Wolfensberger, May 26, 1983, English Translation of Interview with Wolfensberger in *Klik*, May 1983, Wolf Wolfensberger Collection, University of Nebraska Medical Center Archives; Wolfensberger, "Contribution to the History," 74.

70. Wolfensberger, "Contribution to the History," 88.

71. Scull, Andrew T., *Decarceration: Community Treatment and the Deviant: A Radical View* (Englewood Cliffs, NJ: Prentice-Hall, 1977); Grob, Gerald N., *From Asylum to Community: Mental Health Policy in Modern America* (Princeton, NJ: Princeton University Press, 1991); Wolfensberger, "Contribution to the History," 93–94.

72. Zigler, Edward, and Sally J. Styfco, *The Hidden History of Head Start* (Oxford, UK: Oxford University Press, 2010).

73. Zigler, Edward, "Familial Mental Retardation: A Continuing Dilemma," *Science* 155, no. 3760 (1967): 292–98.

74. Zigler (1976) quoted in Hodapp, Robert M., and Edward Zigler, "Integration and Development: Reconciling Two Conflicting Perspectives," *McGill Journal of Education* 27, no. 3 (1992): 279–92, 281.

75. Zigler, Edward, Robert M. Hodapp, and Mark R. Edison, "From Theory to Practice in the Care and Education of Mentally Retarded Individuals," *American Journal on Mental Retardation* 95, no. 1 (1990): 1–12, 7.

76. Zigler et al., "From Theory to Practice"; Blatt, Burton, and Fred Kaplan, *Christmas in Purgatory: A Photographic Essay on Mental Retardation* (Boston: Allyn and Bacon, 1966); Crissey, Marie Skodak, and Marvin Rosen, eds., *Institutions for the Mentally Retarded: A Changing Role in Changing Times* (Austin, TX: Pro-Ed, 1986), 171–78.

77. Greenspan, Stephen, and Mary Cerreto, "Normalization, Deinstitutionalization, and the Limits of Research: Comment on Landesman and Butterfield," *American Psychologist* 44, no. 2 (1989): 448–49, 448.

78. Ramey, Sharon Landesman, "Staging (and Re-Staging) the Trio of Services, Evaluation, and Research," *American Journal on Mental Retardation* 95, no. 1 (1990): 26–29, 27.

79. Wolfensberger, Wolf, "Research, Empiricism, and the Principle of Normalization," in *Normalization, Social Integration and Community Services*, ed. Robert J. Flynn and Kathleen E. Nitsch, 117–29 (Austin, TX: Pro-Ed, 1980), 124–25.

80. Wolfensberger, "Research, Empiricism," 125; Hodapp, Robert M., and Edward Zigler, "Integration and Development: Reconciling Two Conflicting Perspectives," *McGill Journal of Education* 27, no. 3 (1992): 279–92, 280.

81. Hodapp, Robert M., and Elisabeth M. Dykens, "Mental Retardation's Two Cultures of Behavioral Research," *American Journal on Mental Retardation* 98, no. 6 (1994):

675–87; Dykens, Elisabeth M., "Measuring Behavioral Phenotypes: Provocations From the 'New Genetics,'" *American Journal on Mental Retardation* 99, no. 5 (1995): 522–32; Hogan, Andrew J., *Life Histories of Genetic Disease: Patterns and Prevention in Postwar Medical Genetics* (Baltimore: Johns Hopkins University Press, 2016); Hogan, "'Two Cultures' in Clinical Psychology."

82. Schmidt, *Eradicating Deafness?*, 107–32; Navon, Daniel, *Mobilizing Mutations: Human Genetics in the Age of the Patient* (Chicago: University of Chicago Press, 2019).

83. Seligman, Martin E, and Mihaly Csikszentmihalyi, "Positive Psychology: An Introduction," *American Psychologist* 55, no. 1 (2000): 5–14.

84. Elisabeth Dykens, interview with author, May 5, 2017; *Mental Retardation: Definition, Classification, and Systems of Supports*, 9th ed. (Washington, DC: American Association on Mental Retardation, 1992).

85. Dykens, Elisabeth M., "Toward a Positive Psychology of Mental Retardation," *American Journal of Orthopsychiatry* 76, no. 2 (2006): 185–93, 185.

86. Dykens, "Toward a Positive Psychology," 189.

87. Seligman and Csikszentmihalyi, "Positive Psychology"; Hart, Kenneth E., and Thomas Sasso, "Mapping the Contours of Contemporary Positive Psychology," *Canadian Psychology* 52, no. 2 (2011): 82–92, 90–91; Shogren, Karrie A., "Positive Psychology and Disability: A Historical Analysis," in *The Oxford Handbook of Positive Psychology*, ed. Michael L. Wehmeyer, 19–35 (New York: Oxford University Press, 2013), 21; Dunn, Dana S., Gitendra Uswatte, Timothy R. Elliott, Alissa Lastres, and Brittany Beard, "A Positive Psychology of Physical Disability: Principles and Progress," in *The Oxford Handbook of Positive Psychology*, ed. Michael L. Wehmeyer, 427–41 (New York: Oxford University Press, 2013), 441.

88. Stapp, Joy, and Robert Fulcher, "The Employment of APA Members: 1982," *American Psychologist* 38, no. 12 (1983): 1298–320; Lin, Luona, Karen Stamm, and Peggy Christidis, *Demographics of the US Psychology Workforce: Findings From the 2007–16 American Community Survey* (Washington, DC: American Psychological Association, 2018); Andrews et al., "#SaytheWord."

89. Wright, "Spread in Adjustment to Disability"; Andrews, interview.

Chapter 2. Pediatrics

1. Margaret J. Giannini, interview with Eileen M. Oullette, March 8, 2007, Gartner Pediatric History Center, Oral History Project, American Academy of Pediatrics, https://downloads.aap.org/AAP/Gartner%20Pediatric%20History/Giannini_Margaret_Oral_History.pdf.

2. Giannini, interview.

3. Giannini, interview.

4. Thelander, Hulda E., "Programming for Children with Brain Deficit," June 30, 1959, 6, Hulda E. Thelander Papers (HT), North Baker Research Library, California Historical Society (CHS); "Child Development Program at Children's Hospital: Fact Sheet for Occupational Therapy Students," September 23, 1955, 3 (HT, CHS); Strother, C. R., "A Proposal for the Establishment of a Center for Mentally Retarded Children at the University of Washington," October 1962, 15, Proposal for Establishment of Center at UW, 1962–63

Folder, Box 1, acc88–031, UW Child Development and Mental Retardation Center Records (CDMRC), University of Washington Archives (UW).

5. "Annual Report of the Committee on the Handicapped Child, 1956," 15–16, Committee on Children with Disabilities Collection (CCWD), American Academy of Pediatrics Archive (AAP).

6. Knobloch, Hilda, "Teaching Mental Retardation in Medical Education, September 1957," 3, Committee on the Handicapped Child (American Academy of Pediatrics) Folder, Box 119A3, Robert E. Cooke Collection (RC), Alan Mason Chesney Medical Archives of the Johns Hopkins Medical Institutions (JHMI); Koch, Richard, and Kathryn Jean Koch, *Understanding the Mentally Retarded Child: A New Approach* (New York: Random House, 1974), 210; Abbott, Andrew, *The System of Professions: An Essay on the Division of Expert Labor* (Chicago: University of Chicago Press, 1988).

7. Olshansky, Simon, and Leon Sternfeld, "Attitudes of Some Pediatricians toward the Institutionalization of Mentally Retarded Children," *Training School Bulletin* 59, no. 1 (1962): 67–73; Arnhold, Rainer G., and Evelyn R. Callas, "Composition of a Suburban Pediatric Office Practice: An Analysis of Patient Visits during One Year," *Clinical Pediatrics* 5, no. 12 (1966): 722–27.

8. Noll, Steven, and James W. Trent, *Mental Retardation in America: A Historical Reader* (New York: New York University Press, 2004), especially pages 130–64 and 322–83. Vicedo, Marga, *Intelligent Love: The Story of Clara Park, Her Autistic Daughter, and the Myth of the Refrigerator Mother* (Boston: Beacon Press, 2021).

9. Powers, Grover F., "John Howland Award Address," *Pediatrics* 12, no. 2 (1953): 217–26, 219.

10. Park, Edwards A., John W. Littlefield, Henry M. Seidel, and Lawrence S. Wissow, *The Harriet Lane Home: A Model and a Gem* (Baltimore: Johns Hopkins University, 2006), 252–53.

11. Powers, "John Howland Award Address," 224; Cooke, Robert E., "Developmental of Mental Retardation Training Facilities in Medical Schools, May 1962," Box 119D6 (RC, JHMI).

12. Powers, "John Howland Award Address," 225.

13. Carey, Allison C., *On the Margins of Citizenship: Intellectual Disability and Civil Rights in Twentieth-Century America* (Philadelphia: Temple University Press, 2009), 120–25; Castles, Katherine, "'Nice Average Americans': Postwar Parents' Groups and the Defense of the Normal Family," in *Mental Retardation in America: A Historical Reader*, ed. Steven Noll and James W. Trent, 351–70 (New York: New York University Press, 2004); Wright, David, *Downs: The History of a Disability* (New York: Oxford University Press, 2011); Nielsen, Kim E., *A Disability History of the United States* (Boston: Beacon Press, 2012).

14. Munns, George F., "Committee on Mentally and Physically Handicapped Children, August 1955 Report" (CCWD, AAP).

15. Beaven, Paul W., "Adoption of Handicapped Children," *Pediatrics* 17, no. 6 (1956): 970–71, 971.

16. Denhoff, Eric, "Committee on Mentally and Physically Handicapped Children, February 7, 1956 Report" (CCWD, AAP).

17. Beaven, Paul W., "The Adoption of Retarded Children," *Child Welfare* 35, no. 4 (1956): 20–22, 21.

18. Beaven, "Adoption of Handicapped Children," 970.

19. Christopherson, E. H., "Minutes of the Executive Board Meeting, October 1958," 147 (CCWD, AAP).

20. Denhoff, Eric, "Minutes: Committee on the Handicapped Child, October 17, 1960," 2 (CCWD, AAP); "Executive Board Meeting," *American Academic of Pediatrics Newsletter* 11, no. 4 (May 1960): 1–3, 2, American Academy of Pediatrics Newsletter Collection (AAP).

21. Kugel, Robert, "Memorandum, November 20, 1961" (HT, CHS).

22. Kugel, "Memorandum"; Harry A. Waisman to Robert Kugel, November 7, 1961 (HT, CHS).

23. Auerbach, Victor H., Harry A. Waisman, and L. Benjamin Wyckoff, "Phenylketonuria in the Rat associated with Decreased Temporal Discrimination Learning," *Nature* 182, no. 4639 (1958): 871–72; Paul, Diane B., and Jeffrey P. Brosco, *The PKU Paradox: A Short History of a Genetic Disease* (Baltimore: Johns Hopkins University Press, 2013).

24. Waisman to Kugel, November 7, 1961 (HT, CHS).

25. Collett, Robert W., "National Association for Retarded Children, Inc (NARC), Liaison Representative Report, October 1961" (CCWD, AAP).

26. Shorter, Edward, *The Kennedy Family and the Story of Mental Retardation* (Philadelphia: Temple University Press, 2000).

27. Robert Sargent Shriver Jr. to Thomas B. Turner, December 23, 1959, General, 1959–1970 Folder, Box 119B3 (RC, JHMI); Park et al., *Harriet Lane Home*, 268–69.

28. Wallace, Weldon, "Hopkins Studying Causes of Mental Retardation," *Baltimore Sun*, March 8 1958, 16, Cooke Biography Folder, Articles About, 4 (RC, JHMI).

29. Robert E. Cooke, interview by Robert Grayson, September 8, 1996, Oral History Project, Pediatric History Center, American Academy of Pediatrics, https://downloads .aap.org/AAP/Gartner%20Pediatric%20History/Cooke.pdf; Robert E. Cooke to Hollis Huston, March 22, 1967, Correspondence 512 652 H Folder (RC, JHMI); Gauer, Neil A., "Triumph amid the Tumult," Cooke Biography Folder, Articles About, 5 (RC, JHMI); Weber, Bruce, "Robert Cooke, Pediatrician Who Helped Create Head Start, Dies at 93," *New York Times*, February 10, 2014.

30. Robert E. Cooke to Robert Sargent Shriver Jr., November 11, 1959, General, 1959–1970 Folder, Box 119B3 (RC, JHMI).

31. Robert E. Cooke, interview by John F. Stewart, March 29, 1968, 21, John F. Kennedy Library Oral History Program, https://www.jfklibrary.org/sites/default/files /archives/JFKOH/Cooke%2C%20Robert%20E/JFKOH-REC-01/JFKOH-REC-01-TR.pdf; Gauer, "Triumph amid the Tumult."

32. Cooke, interview by Stewart, 5–6.

33. Cooke, Robert E., "Freedom from Handicap," August 26, 1962, 22, Speeches, Seattle Folder, Box 119E1 (RC, JHMI).

34. Cooke, Robert E., "Two Years, Ten Months, and Two Days of Accomplishment on Behalf of the Handicapped," November 25, 1963, 13, Speeches, Dallas Folder, Box 119E2 (RC, JHMI).

35. Cooke, "Two Years," 15.

36. Thelander, Hulda E., "Programming for Children with Brain Deficit," June 30, 1959, 6 (HT, CHS); "Child Development Program at Children's Hospital: Fact Sheet for Occupational Therapy Students," September 23, 1955, 3 (HT, CHS); Strother, "Proposal for the Establishment," 15.

37. Collett, "NARC Liaison Report," 2.

38. Carey, *On the Margins of Citizenship*, 120–25; Castles, "Nice Average Americans."

39. Fenton, Thomas T., "Retardation Shift Urged," *Baltimore Sun* [*Sunday*], October 13, 1963, Cooke Biography Folder, Articles About, 1 (RC, JHMI).

40. Fenton, Thomas T., "Retardation Transfer Hit," *Baltimore Sun* [*Sunday*], October 27, 1963, 24, 512 659 MR MD Facilities Folder (RC, JHMI).

41. Koch and Koch, *Understanding the Mentally Retarded Child*, 210.

42. Denhoff, Eric, "Committee on the Handicapped Child Report," July 1958, 2 (CCWD, AAP).

43. Thelander, "Programming for Children with Brain Deficit," 6 (HT, CHS); Robert Warner to Hulda E. Thelander, August 26, 1960, 1 (HT, CHS).

44. Strother, "Proposal for the Establishment."

45. Association of University Affiliated Facilities (AUAF), "Membership List—Revised Oct 18, 1973," UAF 1971, 1972 Folder, Box 5 (CDMRC, UW).

46. AUAF Annual Meeting Program, May 15–16, 1972, UAF Newsletter Info Folder, Box 4 (CDMRC, UW).

47. Long Range Planning Task Force Folder, Box 119D2 (RC, JHMI); Robert E. Cooke to Eunice Kennedy Shriver, September 21, 1964, E K Shriver, 431 966 388 Folder (RC, JHMI); Farlee, Coralie, "Draft Chapter: History of the Long Range Planning Task Force," January 1976, 6–7; George Tarjan, interview by Milton J. E. Senn, April 24, 1978, 1–5, Oral History of the American Child Guidance Clinical and Child Psychiatry Movement in the USA, National Library of Medicine Archives.

48. Committee on Children with Handicaps, *The Pediatrician and the Child with Mental Retardation* (Evanston, IL: American Academy of Pediatrics, 1971), i–ii.

49. Solomons, Gerald, and Frank J. Menolascino, "Medical Counseling of Parents of the Retarded: The Importance of a Right Start," *Clinical Pediatrics* 7, no. 1 (1968): 11–16, 11–12.

50. American Medical Association, "Mental Retardation: A Handbook for the Primary Physician," *JAMA* 191, no. 3 (1965): 183–222, 191–92, 208.

51. Pearson, Paul H., "The Physician's Role in Diagnosis and Management of the Mentally Retarded," *Pediatric Clinics of North America* 15, no. 4 (1968): 835–59, 837–38.

52. Koch, Richard, Betty V. Graliker, Russell Sands, and Arthur H Parmelee, "Attitude Study of Parents with Mentally Retarded Children: I. Evaluation of Parental Satisfaction with the Medical Care of a Retarded Child," *Pediatrics* 23, no. 3 (1959): 582–84, 583; Waskowitz, Charlotte H., "The Parents of Retarded Children Speak for Themselves," *Journal of Pediatrics* 54, no. 3 (1959): 319–29, 323.

53. John C. Carey, interview by author, August 12, 2019.

54. Committee on the Handicapped Child, "Minutes of Meeting," April 1968, 1 (CCWD, AAP).

55. Committee on Children with Handicaps, *Pediatrician and the Child*, i–ii.

56. Committee on Children with Handicaps, *Pediatrician and the Child*, 10–11.

57. Battle, Constance U., "The Role of the Pediatrician as Ombudsman in the Health Care of the Young Handicapped Child," *Pediatrics* 50, no. 6 (1972): 916–22, 916–17; "Changing the Face of Medicine: Dr. Constance Elizabeth Urciolo Battle," US National Library of Medicine, https://cfmedicine.nlm.nih.gov/physicians/biography_27.html.

58. Battle, "Role of the Pediatrician as Ombudsman, 916–17.

59. Kanthor, Harold, Barry Pless, Betty Satterwhite, and Gary Myers, "Areas of Responsibility in the Health Care of Multiply Handicapped Children," *Pediatrics* 54, no. 6 (1974): 779–85, 784.

60. Pueschel, Siegfried M., and Ann Murphy, "Counseling Parents of Infants with Down's Syndrome," *Postgraduate Medicine* 58, no. 7 (1975): 90–95, 90–91.

61. Pueschel, Siegfried M., *The Young Child with Down Syndrome* (New York: Human Sciences Press, 1984); Pueschel, Siegfried M., *A Parent's Guide to Down Syndrome: Toward a Brighter Future* (Baltimore: Paul H. Brookes, 1990).

62. Carey, *On the Margins of Citizenship*, 146–47.

63. Palfrey, Judith S., Richard C. Mervis, and John A. Butler, "New Directions in the Evaluation and Education of Handicapped Children," *New England Journal of Medicine* 298, no. 15 (1978): 819–24, 820.

64. Jacobs, Francine H., and Deborah Kline Walker, "Pediatricians and the Education for All Handicapped Children Act of 1975 (Public Law 94-142)," *Pediatrics* 61, no. 1 (1978): 135–37, 136.

65. Committee on Children with Handicaps Minutes, April 1976, 8 (CCWD, AAP).

66. Committee on Children with Handicaps Minutes, November 1976, 3; Committee on Children with Handicaps Annual Report, June 1977, 1 (CCWD, AAP).

67. Committee on Children with Handicaps Minutes, April 1977, 4 (CCWD, AAP).

68. Joint Meeting of the Committee on the Handicapped Child and the Committee on Mental Retardation of the Section on Child Development, October 1966, 6; Committee on the Handicapped Child, "Minutes of Meeting," April 1968, 5–6 (CCWD, AAP).

69. Committee on Children with Handicaps Minutes, April 1977, 4 (CCWD, AAP).

70. Committee on Children with Handicaps Minutes, October 1977, 12 (CCWD, AAP).

71. Denhoff, Eric, "Education for the Child with Handicaps: Current Status," May 1980" (CCWD, AAP).

72. Committee on Children with Handicaps Minutes, April 1978, 1; Committee on Children with Handicaps Minutes, June 1980, 18 (CCWD, AAP).

73. Committee on Children with Handicaps Minutes, November 1980, 4 (CCWD, AAP).

74. Koch and Koch, *Understanding the Mentally Retarded*, 37–38; Committee on Children with Handicaps Minutes, November 1978, 2 (CCWD, AAP).

75. Antommaria, Armand Matheny, "*Who Should Survive? One of the Choices on Our Conscience*: Mental Retardation and the History of Contemporary Bioethics," *Kennedy Institute of Ethics Journal* 16, no. 3 (2006): 205–24.

76. Cooke, Robert E., "Whose Suffering," *Journal of Pediatrics* 80, no. 5 (1972): 906–8; Cooke, Robert E., "The Role of Ethics in Pediatrics," *American Journal of Diseases of Children* 129, no. 10 (1975): 1157–61; Cooke, Robert E., "Ethics on Behalf of the Mentally Retarded," *Pediatric Annals* 10 (1981): 24–30.

77. Committee on Children with Handicaps Minutes, March 1983, Attachment 2 (CCWD, AAP).

78. Wright, *Downs*, 161–64.

79. Haggerty, Robert J., "The Changing Role of the Pediatrician in Child Health Care," *American Journal of Diseases of Children* 127, no. 4 (1974): 545–49, 547.

80. Council on Pediatric Practice, *Standards of Child Health Care* (Evanston, IL: American Academy of Pediatrics, 1967), 77.

81. Sia, Calvin C., "Abraham Jacobi Award Address, April 14, 1992, The Medical Home: Pediatric Practice and Child Advocacy in the 1990s," *Pediatrics* 90, no. 3 (1992): 419–23, 420.

82. Sia, Calvin, Thomas F. Tonniges, Elizabeth Osterhus, and Sharon Taba, "History of the Medical Home Concept," *Pediatrics* 113, no. 5 (2004): 1473–78, 1473–74; Calvin C. Sia, interview with author, June 27, 2019.

83. Battle, "Role of the Pediatrician," 921; Kanthor et al., "Areas of Responsibility."

84. Committee on Children with Disabilities Minutes, November 1988, 8 (CCWD, AAP); Ad Hoc Task Force on Definition of the Medical Home, "The Medical Home," *Pediatrics* 90, no. 5 (1992): 774.

85. Ad Hoc Task Force, "Medical Home," 774.

86. Committee on Children with Disabilities, "Care Coordination: Integrating Health and Related Systems of Care for Children with Special Health Care Needs," *Pediatrics* 104, no. 4 (1999): 978–81, 979. CCWH became CCWD in 1983.

87. Committee on Children with Disabilities Minutes, December 1994, 15 (CCWD, AAP).

88. Committee on Children with Disabilities Minutes, May 1994, 24 (CCWD, AAP).

89. Committee on Children with Disabilities Minutes, December 1994, 2 (CCWD, AAP).

90. Committee on Children with Disabilities Minutes, November 2000, 12 (CCWD, AAP); Committee on Children with Disabilities Minutes, March 2001, 10 (CCWD, AAP).

91. Committee on Child Health Financing, *The Medical Home for Children: Financing Principles* (American Academy of Pediatrics, 2012), 8, https://medicalhomeinfo.aap.org /tools-resources/Documents/MHfinanceprin.pdf.

92. Cooley, W. Carl, and Committee on Children with Disabilities, "Providing a Primary Care Medical Home for Children and Youth with Cerebral Palsy," *Pediatrics* 114, no. 4 (2004): 1106–13, 1108.

93. Homer, Charles J. et al., "A Review of the Evidence for the Medical Home for Children with Special Health Care Needs," *Pediatrics* 122, no. 4 (2008): e922–37; Homer, Charles J., W. Carl Cooley, and Bonnie Strickland, "Medical Home 2009: What It Is, Where We Were, and Where We Are Today," *Pediatric Annals* 38, no. 9 (2009): 483–90, 483.

94. Zola, Irving K., "Toward the Necessary Universalizing of a Disability Policy," *Milbank Quarterly* 67, Supplement 2, Part 2 (1989): 401–28.

95. Amy J. Houtrow, interview by author, October 23, 2019.

Chapter 3. Genetic Counseling

1. Marks, Joan H., "The Training of Genetic Counselors: Origins of a Psychosocial Model," in *Prescribing Our Future: Ethical Challenges in Genetic Counseling*, ed. Dianne M.

Bartels, Bonnie S. LeRoy, and Arthur L. Caplan, 15–24 (New York: Aldine de Gruyter, 1993), 18.

2. Laura Hercher, interview with author, August 16, 2018.

3. Stern, Alexandra Minna, *Telling Genes: The Story of Genetic Counseling in America* (Baltimore: Johns Hopkins University Press, 2012); Stillwell, Devon, "'Pretty Pioneering-Spirited People': Genetic Counsellors, Gender Culture, and the Professional Evolution of a Feminised Health Field, 1947–1980," *Social History of Medicine* 28, no. 1 (2015): 172–93.

4. Kenen, Regina H., "Genetic Counseling: The Development of a New Interdisciplinary Occupational Field," *Social Science and Medicine* 18, no. 7 (1984): 541–49, 546.

5. Stern, *Telling Genes*; Stillwell, "Pretty Pioneering-Spirited People"; Comfort, Nathaniel, *The Science of Human Perfection: Heredity and Health in American Biomedicine* (New Haven, CT: Yale University Press, 2012).

6. Lippman, Abby, and Benjamin S. Wilfond, "Twice-Told Tales: Stories about Genetic Disorders," *American Journal of Human Genetics* 51, no. 4 (1992): 936–37; Wertz, Dorothy C., "What's Missing from Genetic Counseling: A Survey of 476 Counseling Sessions," *Journal of Genetic Counseling* 7, no. 6 (1998): 499–500; Kline, Laura, "Disability Awareness Training and Implications for Current Practice: A Survey of Genetic Counselors" (master's thesis, Brandeis University, 2012); Reed, Amy R., "Genetic Counseling, Professional Values, and Habitus: An Analysis of Disability Narratives in Textbooks," *Journal of Medical Humanities* 39, no. 4 (2018): 515–33; Janice G. Edwards, interview with author, August 6, 2019; Kathryn F. Peters, interview with author, July 31, 2018.

7. Kessler, Seymour, "The Psychological Paradigm Shift in Genetic Counseling," *Social Biology* 27, no. 3 (1980): 167–85, 182.

8. Anabel Stenzel graduated from the genetic counseling master's program at the University of California, Berkeley in 1997. She worked for sixteen years at Stanford University Children's Hospital. Stenzel had cystic fibrosis and received two double-lung transplants during her lifetime. She died of cancer in 2013. Byrnes, Isabel Stenzel, and Anabel Stenzel, *The Power of Two: A Twin Triumph Over Cystic Fibrosis* (Columbia: University of Missouri Press, 2007). PhD biologist Judith Tsipis founded and directed the Brandeis University genetic counseling training program, beginning in 1992. Tsipis had a son with disabilities, and oriented the Brandeis program around greater disability awareness (chapter 6). Joan Burns, who held master's degrees in genetics and social work, was the first director of the University of Wisconsin–Madison genetic counseling training program. She had a child with "severe" developmental disabilities. Stern, *Telling Genes*, 96; Judith Tsipis, interview with author, July 23, 2018.

9. Stern, Alexandra Minna, "A Quiet Revolution: The Birth of the Genetic Counselor at Sarah Lawrence College, 1969," *Journal of Genetic Counseling* 18, no. 1 (2009): 1–11, 3.

10. Marks, "Training of Genetic Counselors," 19–20.

11. Epstein, Charles J., "Who Should Do Genetic Counseling, and Under What Circumstances?," *Birth Defects Original Article Series* 9, no. 4 (1973): 39–48, 44.

12. Marks, Joan H., and Melissa L. Richter, "The Genetic Associate: A New Health Professional," *American Journal of Public Health* 66, no. 4 (1976): 388–90.

13. Kenen, "Genetic Counseling," 544.

14. Heimler, Audrey, "An Oral History of the National Society of Genetic Counselors," *Journal of Genetic Counseling* 6, no. 3 (1997): 315–36, 320.

15. Audrey Heimler, communication with author, August 5, 2020.

16. Epstein, Charles J., "Foreword," in *Genetic Counseling: Psychological Dimensions*, ed. Seymour Kessler, xv–xix (New York: Academic Press, 1979), xvii.

17. Heimler, "Oral History," 317.

18. Epstein, "Foreword," xix.

19. Hochschild, Arlie Russell, *The Managed Heart: Commercialization of Human Feeling* (Berkeley: University of California Press, 1983); Stern, *Telling Genes*, 122.

20. Bosk, Charles, *All God's Mistakes: Genetic Counseling in a Pediatric Hospital* (Chicago: University of Chicago Press, 1992), 57–82.

21. Robert G. Resta, interview with author, May 17, 2019.

22. Robin L. Bennett, interview with author, May 17, 2019; Stillwell, "Pretty Pioneering-Spirited People."

23. Bonnie S. LeRoy, interview with author, November 9, 2018.

24. LeRoy, interview; Mark S. Lubinski, interview with author, July 16, 2019.

25. Deborah L. Eunpu, interview with author, May 16, 2018; Barbara B. Biesecker, interview with author, July 25, 2018; Stillwell, "Pretty Pioneering-Spirited People."

26. Bennett, interview.

27. Bay, Carolyn, "Parent Groups: A Mechanism to Facilitate Parental Adjustment, and a Useful Addition to the Genetic Counseling Team," *Perspectives in Genetic Counseling* 1, no. 2 (1979): 1–2, 1; *Perspectives in Genetic Counseling* available at: https://www.nsgc.org/page/perspectives.

28. Fine, Beth A., "Resources," *Perspectives in Genetic Counseling* 4, no. 1 (1982): 3.

29. Fine, Beth A., "Resources: Developmental Disabilities Services," *Perspectives in Genetic Counseling* 4, no. 4 (1982): 4–5, 5.

30. Mark S. Lubinsky, interview with author, July 16, 2019.

31. Resta, interview.

32. Halperin, Dorothy, "Review of *Trisomy 18: A Book for Families*," *Perspectives in Genetic Counseling* 6, no. 1 (1984): 1.

33. Baty, Bonnie Jeanne, "Correspondence: To the Editor," *Perspectives in Genetic Counseling* 6, no. 3 (1984): 5–6, 5.

34. Kelly E. Ormond, interview with author, February 26, 2019; Greendale, Karen, "Beth Fine Kaplan—Colleague and Friend," *Journal of Genetic Counseling* 7, no. 5 (1998): 381–83.

35. Kirschner, Kristi L., Kelly E. Ormond, and Carol J. Gill, "The Impact of Genetic Technologies on Perceptions of Disability," *Quality Management in Health Care* 8, no. 3 (2000): 19–26.

36. Saxton, Marsha, "Born and Unborn: The Implications of Genetic Technologies for People with Disabilities," in *Test-Tube Women: What Future for Motherhood?*, ed. Rita Arditti, Renate Duelli Klein, and Shelley Minden, 298–312 (London: Pandora Press, 1984); Asch, Adrienne, "The Human Genome and Disability Rights: Thoughts for Researchers and Advocates," *Disability Studies Quarterly* 13, no. 3 (1993): 3–4.

37. Hubbard, Ruth, "A Feminist Views Prenatal Diagnosis," *Perspectives in Genetic Counseling* 10, no. 2 (1988): 1–12, 12.

38. Saxton, Marsha, "Rights of the Disabled: A Message to Professionals," *Perspectives in Genetic Counseling* 10, no. 2 (1988): 1–4, 4.

39. Marks, Joan H., and Seymour Kessler, "To the Editor, PGC: No Place for Ideology," *Perspectives in Genetic Counseling* 10, no. 3 (1988): 5.

40. Marks, "Training of Genetic Counselors"; Kessler, "Psychological Paradigm Shift."

41. Brasington, Campbell K., "What I Wish I Knew Then . . . Reflections from Personal Experiences in Counseling about Down Syndrome," *Journal of Genetic Counseling* 16 (2007): 731–34, 731.

42. Epstein, Charles J. et al., "Genetic Counseling," *American Journal of Human Genetics* 27, no. 2 (1975): 240–42.

43. National Society of Genetic Counselors, "Genetic Counselor Description," *Perspectives in Genetic Counseling* 5, no. 4 (1983): 3.

44. Faucett, Andrew, "Letters to the Editor: Finding Funding Support," *Perspectives in Genetic Counseling* 14, no. 3 (1992): 11; Weinblatt, Vivian J., "Letters to the Editor: Professional Roles vs. Personal Beliefs," *Perspectives in Genetic Counseling* 15, no. 1 (1993): 14.

45. Magyari, Trish, and Robin Belsky Gold, "Social Issues: Membership Defined by Committee Survey Resultsb" *Perspectives in Genetic Counseling* 10, no. 4 (1988): 1–4, 4.

46. McConkie-Rosell, Allyn, and Dorene Markel, "Facilitating Research: The Many Roles of the Genetic Counselor," *Perspectives in Genetic Counseling* 17, no. 2 (1995): 1–4, 1; Benkendorf, Judith L., "To the Editor: Challenges for Genetic Counselors in Research Roles," *Perspectives in Genetic Counseling* 17, no. 3 (1995): 13.

47. Langfelder, Elinor, "Letters to the Editor: A World without Genetic Counselors?," *Perspectives in Genetic Counseling* 16, no. 4 (1994): 8.

48. Biesecker, Barbara B., and Kathryn F. Peters, "Process Studies in Genetic Counseling: Peering into the Black Box," *American Journal of Medical Genetics* 106, no. 3 (2001): 191–98; National Society of Genetic Counselors' Definition Task Force, "A New Definition of Genetic Counseling: National Society of Genetic Counselors' Task Force Report," *Journal of Genetic Counseling* 15, no. 2 (2006): 77–83.

49. Gorlin, Rena A., *Codes of Professional Responsibility*, 2nd ed. (Washington, DC: Bureau of National Affairs, 1990), 179–288; Benkendorf, Judith L., Nancy P. Callanan, Rose Grobstein, Susan Schmerler, and Kevin T. FitzGerald, "An Explication of the National Society of Genetic Counselors (NSGC) Code of Ethics," *Journal of Genetic Counseling* 1, no. 1 (1992): 31–39; Ormond, interview; Bennett, interview.

50. Benkendorf et al., "Explication of the NSGC Code of Ethics," 39.

51. Grobstein, Rose, and Judith Benkendorf, "Our Code of Ethics: Society and You," *Perspectives in Genetic Counseling* 16, no. 2 (1994): 11.

52. Mittman, Ilana, Stephanie Smith, and Colleen Dougherty, "Encouraging Diversity among Genetic Counselors," *Perspectives in Genetic Counseling* 17, no. 3 (1995): 1–7, 7; Mittman, Ilana S., and Katy Downs, "Diversity in Genetic Counseling: Past, Present and Future," *Journal of Genetic Counseling* 17, no. 4 (2008): 301–13, 305; Bao, Annie K., Amanda L. Bergner, Gayun Chan-Smutko, and Janelle Villiers, "Reflections on Diversity, Equity, and Inclusion in Genetic Counseling Education," *Journal of Genetic Counseling* 29, no. 2 (2020): 315–23.

53. Senter, Leigha et al., "National Society of Genetic Counselors Code of Ethics: Explication of 2017 Revisions." *Journal of Genetic Counseling* 27, no. 1 (2018): 9–15.

54. Greendale, Karen, "Message from Your President," *Perspectives in Genetic Counseling* 15, no. 4 (1993): 2.

55. "Point Counterpoint: Do We Support the Restructuring of ABMG?," *Perspectives in Genetic Counseling* 14, no. 3 (1992): 8–9, 8.

56. Kessler, Seymour, *Genetic Counseling: Psychological Dimensions* (New York: Academic Press, 1979), 57.

57. Blatt, Robin J. R., *Prenatal Tests: What They Are, Their Benefits and Risks, and How to Decide Whether to Have Them or Not* (New York: Vintage, 1988), 191; Kessler, Seymour, "Psychological Aspects of Genetic Counseling: VII. Thoughts on Directiveness," *Journal of Genetic Counseling* 1, no. 1 (1992): 9–17; Fine, Beth A., "The Evolution of Nondirectiveness in Genetic Counseling and Implications of the Human Genome Project," in *Prescribing Our Future: Ethical Challenges in Genetic Counseling*, ed. Dianne M. Bartels, Bonnie S. LeRoy, and Arthur L. Caplan, 101–18 (New York: Aldine de Gruyter, 1993), 115; Bendor, Linda Whipperman, "Nondirectiveness: Defining Our Goals and Methods," *Perspectives in Genetic Counseling* 18, no. 4 (1996): 1–9, 1; Veach, Patricia McCarthy, Dianne M. Bartels, and Bonnie S. LeRoy, "Commentary on Genetic Counseling: A Profession in Search of Itself," *Journal of Genetic Counseling* 11, no. 3 (2002): 187–91; Weil, Jon, "Psychosocial Genetic Counseling in the Post-Nondirective Era: A Point of View," *Journal of Genetic Counseling* 12, no. 3 (2003): 199–211.

58. R. Stephen Amato, interview with author, May 2, 2018; John C. Carey, interview with author, August 12, 2019.

59. Virginia L. Corson, interview with author, July 10, 2018; Brenda Finucane, interview with author, June 7, 2018.

60. LeRoy, interview.

61. Biesecker, interview.

62. Ellyn Farrelly, interview with author, February 26, 2019.

63. Dinnen, Rich, and Bonnie Hatten, "Masters Level Projects," *Perspectives in Genetic Counseling* 16, no. 2 (1994): 10; Warren, Nancy Steinberg, and Betsy Gettig, "To the Editor: Directors Respond to Comments about Thesis Topics," *Perspectives in Genetic Counseling* 16, no. 3 (1994): 10.

64. Wertz, "What's Missing from Genetic Counseling," 500; Krogh, Jacqueline, and Liz Stierman, "The Buzz from Denver," *Perspectives in Genetic Counseling* 20, no. 4 (1998): 4.

65. Sorenson, James R., "Genetic Counseling: Values That Have Mattered," in *Prescribing Our Future: Ethical Challenges in Genetic Counseling*, ed. Dianne M. Bartels, Bonnie S. Leroy, and Arthur L. Caplan, 3–14 (New York: Aldine de Gruyter, 1993), 11.

66. Finucane, interview.

67. GeneAMP Managed Care Team, "Genetic Counseling Defined by Care," *Perspectives in Genetic Counseling* 19, no. 4 (1997): 4.

68. Benkendorf, Judith L., Helen Travers, and Barbara B. Biesecker, "To the Editor: Second Look Urged for Care Marketing Message," *Perspectives in Genetic Counseling* 20, no. 1 (1998): 7.

69. Managed Care GeneAMP Team, "To the Editor: Response from 'One Voice; One Message' Team," *Perspectives in Genetic Counseling* 20, no. 2 (1998): 8.

70. Margie Goldstein, interview with author, July 18, 2018; Stern, *Telling Genes*, 96–97.

71. Biesecker, interview; Stern, *Telling Genes*, 140–41.

72. Jon Weil, interview with author, July 24, 2018.

73. Weil, interview.

74. Weil, interview; Weil, Jon, *Psychosocial Genetic Counseling* (New York: Oxford University Press, 2000), 262; Rapp, Rayna, *Testing Women, Testing the Fetus: The Social Impact of Amniocentesis in America* (New York: Routledge, 1999), 153–59; Brunger, Fern, and Abby Lippman, "Resistance and Adherence to the Norms of Genetic Counseling," *Journal of Genetic Counseling* 4, no. 3 (1995): 151–67, 160.

75. Weil, *Psychosocial Genetic Counseling*, 259; Beeson, Diane, and Teresa Doksum, "Family Values and Resistance to Genetic Testing," in *Bioethics in Social Context*, ed. Barry Hoffmaster, 153–79 (Philadelphia: Temple University Press, 2001).

76. Weil, *Psychosocial Genetic Counseling*, 270.

77. Weil, *Psychosocial Genetic Counseling*, 267.

78. Weil, interview.

79. Biesecker, interview; "New Training Program," *Perspectives in Genetic Counseling* 17, no. 1 (1995): 14.

80. Biesecker, interview.

81. Biesecker, Barbara B., and Lori Hamby, "What Difference the Disability Community Arguments Should Make for the Delivery of Prenatal Genetic Information," in *Prenatal Testing and Disability Rights*, ed. Erik Parens and Adrienne Asch, 340–57 (Washington, DC: Georgetown University Press, 2000), 351.

82. Lori Hamby Erby, interview with author, March 7, 2019; James, Cynthia, Melissa Barber, Lori Hamby, and Grace-Ann Olayinka, "MDA Camp: Counselors' Experiences," *Perspectives in Genetic Counseling* 21, no. 3 (1999): 1–6.

83. Margie Goldstein, interview with author, July 18, 2018.

84. Schoonveld, K. Cheri, Patricia McCarthy Veach, and Bonnie S. LeRoy, "What Is It Like to Be in the Minority? Ethnic and Gender Diversity in the Genetic Counseling Profession," *Journal of Genetic Counseling* 16, no. 1 (2007): 53–69; Bao, Annie K., Amanda L. Bergner, Gayun Chan-Smutko, and Janelle Villiers, "Reflections on Diversity, Equity, and Inclusion in Genetic Counseling Education," *Journal of Genetic Counseling* 29, no. 2 (2020): 315–23.

Chapter 4. Advocacy before Evidence?

1. On the origins of aversive procedures in autism and continued opposition to behavioral approaches to treatment in autism see: Kirkham, Patrick, "'The Line between Intervention and Abuse': Autism and Applied Behaviour Analysis," *History of the Human Sciences* 30, no. 2 (2017): 107–26; Silberman, Steve, *Neurotribes: The Legacy of Autism and the Future of Neurodiversity* (New York: Avery, 2015); Silverman, Chloe, *Understanding Autism: Patients, Doctors, and the History of a Disorder* (Princeton, NJ: Princeton University Press, 2011).

2. AAMD Position Statement on Aversive Therapy, Official Business of the American Association on Mental Deficiency, 1986–87, 148, American Association on Intellectual and Developmental Disabilities Archives, Silver Spring, MD (AAIDD Archives).

3. AAMD 1975 Statement on Aversives, quoted in: Guess, Doug, Edwin Helmstetter, H. Rutherford Turnbull III, and Suzanne Knowltorr, *Use of Aversive Procedures with Persons Who Are Disabled: An Historical Review and Critical Analysis* (Seattle: Association for Persons with Severe Handicaps, 1987), 29.

4. Trent, James W. Jr., *Inventing the Feeble Mind: A History of Mental Retardation in the United States* (Berkeley: University of California Press, 1994); Gelb, Steven A., "'Mental Deficients' Fighting Fascism: The Unplanned Normalization of World War II," in *Mental Retardation in America: A Historical Reader*, 308–21 (New York: New York University Press, 2004).

5. American Association on Mental Deficiency, Leadership Directories Collection (1954–1999) (AAIDD); David Coulter, interview with author, June 10, 2019.

6. Routh, Donald K., "A History of Division 33 (Psychology in Mental Retardation and Developmental Disabilities)," in *Unification through Division: Histories of the Divisions of the American Psychological Association*, vol. 3, ed. Donald A. Dewsbury, 117–42 (Washington, DC: American Psychological Association, 1999); Silberman, *Neurotribes*.

7. Routh, "History of Division 33," 132–36.

8. Sailor, Wayne, "History of TASH," 2015, https://tash.org/about/history-tash/; Wayne Sailor, interview with author, October 25, 2019.

9. 1981 TASH Executive Committee Resolution on Aversive Procedures, quoted in: Guess et al., *Use of Aversive Procedures*, 29–30 (n. 3).

10. Guess et al., *Use of Aversive Procedures*, 29–30 (n. 3), 1.

11. Sailor, "History of TASH."

12. Matson, Johnny L., "Setting the Record Straight," *AAMR News & Notes* 1, no. 3 (1988): 5. California outlawed the use of aversive interventions as part of the Hughes Act in 1991.

13. Abbott, Andrew, *The System of Professions: An Essay on the Division of Expert Labor* (Chicago: University of Chicago Press, 1988).

14. AAMD Resolution on Publications and Membership Categories, Official Business of AAMD 1986–87, 140 (AAIDD); Gail O'Connor, President's Report, AAMD Report to Council 1982–83, 1–3 (AAIDD); Coulter, interview.

15. Turnbull, H. Rutherford III, "Presidential Address 1986: Public Policy and Professional Behavior," *Mental Retardation* 24, no. 5 (1986): 265–75.

16. Turnbull, Rud. *The Exceptional Life of Jay Turnbull: Disability and Dignity in America 1967–2009* (Amherst, MA: White Poppy Press, 2011), 105.

17. Other major disability advocacy organizations adopted similar position statements calling for the cessation of the use of aversives during the 1980s, including the Association for Retarded Citizens of the United States in 1985 and the Autism Society of America in 1988. Gerhardt, Peter, David L. Holmes, Michael Alessandri, and Michele Goodman, "Social Policy on the Use of Aversive Interventions: Empirical, Ethical, and Legal Considerations," *Journal of Autism and Developmental Disorders* 21, no. 3 (1991): 265–77, 265–66.

18. Keys, Joseph B., "Discussion of Issues Needed," *AAMR News & Notes* 1, no. 3 (1988): 5–8, 8.

19. Linscheid, Thomas, "SIBIS Article Facts Disputed," *AAMR News & Notes* 2, no. 2 (1989): 6.

20. Guess et al., *Use of Aversive Procedures*, 29–30 (n. 3), 31.

21. "AAMR Revises Policy on Aversive Procedures," *AAMR News & Notes* 3, no. 4 (1990): 1.

22. Guess et al., *Use of Aversive Procedures*, 29–30 (n. 3), 32.

23. James A. Mulick, interview with author, April 24, 2019.

24. Mulick, interview; Linscheid, Thomas R., and Charles E. Cunningham, "A Controlled Demonstration of the Effectiveness of Electric Shock in the Elimination of Chronic Infant Rumination," *Journal of Applied Behavior Analysis* 10, no. 3 (1977): 500.

25. Cooke, Robert E., "Whose Suffering," *Journal of Pediatrics* 80, no. 5 (1972): 906–8; Kuhse, Helga, and Peter Singer, "Ethics and the Handicapped Newborn Infant," *Social Research* 52, no. 3 (1985): 505–42; Parens, Erik, and Adrienne Asch, eds., *Prenatal Testing and Disability Rights* (Washington, DC: Georgetown University Press, 2000); Amundson, Ron, and Shari Tresky, "Bioethics and Disability Rights: Conflicting Values and Perspectives," *Journal of Bioethical Inquiry* 5, no. 2 (2008): 111–23; Wilfond, Benjamin S., "Tracheostomies and Assisted Ventilation in Children with Profound Disabilities: Navigating Family and Professional Values," *Pediatrics* 133, Supplement 1 (2014): S44–49; Kukora, Stephanie et al., "Infant with Trisomy 18 and Hypoplastic Left Heart Syndrome," *Pediatrics* 143, no. 5 (2019).

26. Mulick, James A., "The Ideology and Science of Punishment in Mental Retardation," *American Journal of Mental Retardation* 95, no. 2 (1990): 142–56, 142.

27. Mulick, "Ideology and Science of Punishment," 153.

28. Matson, "Setting the Record Straight," (n. 12); Matson, Johnny L., and Naomi B. Swiezy, "The Aversives Controversy: Policy Issues in Behavior Modification and Therapy," *Cognitive Behaviour Therapy* 19, no. 1 (1990): 25–31; Van Houten, Ron et al., "The Right to Effective Behavioral Treatment," *Behavior Analyst* 11, no. 2 (1988): 111–14.

29. Haring, Norris G., and Owen R. White, "Comments on the TASG Monograph and the Mulick Review," *American Journal on Mental Retardation* 95, no. 2 (1990): 163–65, 164.

30. Mulick, James A., and John W. Jacobson, "Some Contingencies Affecting Restrictive Behavioral Interventions," *Psychology in Mental Retardation and Developmental Disabilities* 15, no. 3 (1990): 4–7, 4, Division 33 Collection (Div 33), American Psychological Association Archives (APA).

31. Mulick and Jacobson, "Some Contingencies," 5.

32. Zigler (1976) quoted in Hodapp, Robert M., and Edward Zigler, "Integration and Development: Reconciling Two Conflicting Perspectives," *McGill Journal of Education* 27, no. 3 (1992): 279–92, 281.

33. Jacobson, John W., "Aversive Conditioning: The Jury Is Out," *Psychology in Mental Retardation* 13, no. 3 (1988): 5–7, 7 (Div 33, APA).

34. Wolfensberger, Wolf, "PC: The New Censorship?," *AAMR News & Notes* 4, no. 6 (1991): 2–3.

35. Turnbull, "Presidential Address 1986," 271–72 (n. 14).

36. Michaelson, Robin, "Tug-of-War Is Developing over Defining Retardation," *APA Monitor* May (1993): 34–35, 34 (Div 33, APA).

37. Ruth Luckasson, interview with author, June 12, 2019.

38. Jack Stark, interview with author, January 11, 2019.

39. "Minutes: Division 33, APA Executive Committee Meeting," *Psychology in Mental Retardation* 14, no. 1 (1988): 15 (APA).

40. Coulter, interview.

41. Robert Schalock, interview with author, January 22, 2019.

42. *Mental Retardation: Definition, Classification, and Systems of Supports*, 9th ed. (Washington, DC: American Association on Mental Retardation, 1992), 9.

43. *Mental Retardation*, 1. The ten dimensions were: communication, self-care, social skills, home living, community use, functional academics, health and safety, leisure, work, and self-direction. They were adapted from the special education literature specific to students with moderate to "severe" disabilities. Ford, Alison et al., eds., *The Syracuse Community-Referenced Curriculum Guide for Students with Moderate and Severe Disabilities* (Baltimore: Paul H. Brookes, 1989). For more on the previous system: Grossman, Herbert J., ed., *Classification in Mental Retardation*, 8th ed. (Washington, DC: American Association on Mental Deficiency, 1983).

44. Marc Tassé, interview with author, April 25, 2019.

45. Michaelson, "Tug-of-War Is Developing," 34 (n. 52).

46. Jacobson, John W., and James A. Mulick, "Walkin' the Walk: APA Takes a Step Forward in Professional Practice," *Psychological in Mental Retardation and Developmental Disabilities* 19, no. 1 (1993): 4–8, 6 (Div 33, APA).

47. Michaelson, "Tug-of-War Is Developing" 34 (n. 52).

48. Schalock, interview.

49. Michaelson, "Tug-of-War Is Developing" 34 (n. 52).

50. *Mental Retardation*, 1 (n. 55).

51. Luckasson, interview.

52. Tassé, interview.

53. Macy, Terrence, "MR Definition: Revision Needed," *AAMR News & Notes* 7, no. 3 (1994): 6.

54. Schalock, interview.

55. Coulter, interview.

56. Jacobson, John W., and James A. Mulick, eds., *Manual of Diagnosis and Professional Practice in Mental Retardation* (Washington, DC: American Psychological Association, 1996), 13.

57. Jacobson and Mulick, "Walkin' the Walk," 8 (n. 60); see also: Switzky, Harvey N., and Stephen Greenspan, eds., *What Is Mental Retardation? Ideas for an Evolving Disability in the 21st Century* (Washington, DC: American Association on Mental Retardation, 2006).

58. Tassé, interview.

59. Tassé, interview.

60. "Wolfensberger, Owens, and Wattleton to Address AAMR," *AAMR News & Notes* 5, no. 1 (1992): 3.

61. Van Houten et al., "Right to Effective Behavioral Treatment," (n. 30); Trader, Barb, and Ralph Edwards, "The Continued Debate about Facilitated Communication: A Response From TASH's Executive Director and President of the TASH Board," 2105, https://tash.org/wp-content/uploads/2015/03/FC-Letter.pdf.

62. Biklen, Douglas, *Communication Unbound: How Facilitated Communication Is*

Challenging Traditional Views of Autism and Ability / Disability (New York: Teachers College Press, 1993).

63. Biklen, Douglas, "Communication Unbound: Autism and Praxis," *Harvard Educational Review* 60, no. 3 (1990): 291–314.

64. Biklen, *Communication Unbound*, 47–48.

65. Biklen, *Communication Unbound*, xiii.

66. Biklen, *Communication Unbound*, 184.

67. Cummins, Robert A., and Margot P. Prior, "Further Comment: Autism and Assisted Communication: A Response to Biklen," *Harvard Educational Review* 62, no. 2 (1992): 228–56, 232; Jacobson, John W., Richard M. Foxx, and James A. Mulick, "Facilitated Communication: The Ultimate Fad Treatment," in *Controversial Therapies for Autism and Intellectual Disabilities: Fad, Fashion, and Science in Professional Practice*, 2nd ed., ed. Richard M. Foxx, and James A. Mulick, 283–302 (New York: Routledge, 2015), 284.

68. Biklen, *Communication Unbound*, 59; Stubblefield, Anna, "Sound and Fury: When Opposition to Facilitated Communication Functions as Hate Speech," *Disability Studies Quarterly* 31, no. 4 (2011). Crossley also made a similar argument, comparing the right FC access to hearing aids for deaf children. Crossley, Rosemary, "Talking Politics: Empowering Communication Aid Users," https://www.researchgate.net/publication/266908495 _Talking_Politics_Empowering_Communication_Aid_Users.

69. Cummins and Prior, "Further Comment"; Prior, Margot, and Robert Cummins, "Questions about Facilitated Communication and Autism," *Journal of Autism and Developmental Disorders* 22, no. 3 (1992): 331–38, 336; Heinrichs, Paul, "Experts Slam Disabled Charade," *Sunday Age*, March 10, 1991, 1.

70. Mulick, interview.

71. Szempruch, Joseph, and John W. Jacobson, "Evaluating Facilitated Communications of People with Developmental Disabilities," *Research in Developmental Disabilities* 14, no. 4 (1993): 253–64; Wheeler, Douglas L., John W. Jacobson, Raymond A. Paglieri, and Allen A. Schwaartz, "An Experimental Assessment of Facilitated Communication," *Mental Retardation* 31, no. 1 (1993): 49–60.

72. Biklen, Douglas, and Judith Felson Duchan, "'I Am Intelligent': The Social Construction of Mental Retardation," *Journal of the Association of Persons with Severe Handicaps* 19, no. 3 (1994): 173–84; Williams, Donna, "Invited Commentary: In the Real World," *Journal of the Association for Persons with Severe Handicaps* 19, no. 3 (1994): 196–99.

73. Jacobson, John W., James A. Mulick, and Allen A. Schwartz, "A History of Facilitated Communication: Science, Pseudoscience, and Antiscience," *American Psychologist* 50, no. 9 (1995): 750–65.

74. Jacobson et al., "Facilitated Communication: The Ultimate Fad."

75. Jacobson et al., "History of Facilitated Communication," 752 (n. 91).

76. Jacobson et al., "Facilitated Communication: The Ultimate Fad."

77. Biklen, *Communication Unbound*, 136 (n. 1); Jacobson et al., "History of Facilitated Communication," 759–60.

78. Jacobson, John W., and James A. Mulick, "The Power of Positive Stereotyping, or Have You Changed the Way You Think Yet?," *Psychology in Mental Retardation and Developmental Disabilities* 19, no. 3 (1994): 8–16, 12 (Div 33, APA).

79. Sailor, Wayne, "Science, Ideology, and Facilitated Communication," *American Psychologist* 51, no. 9 (1996): 984–85.

80. Sailor, interview.

81. Margolin, Kenneth N., "How Shall Facilitated Communication Be Judged? Facilitated Communication and the Legal System," in *Facilitated Communication: The Clinical and Social Phenomenon*, ed. Howard C. Shane, 227–58 (San Diego: Singular Publishing Group, 1994); Gorman, Brian J., "Facilitated Communication: Rejected in Science, Accepted in Court: A Case Study and Analysis of the Use of FC Evidence under *Frye* and *Daubert*," *Behavioral Sciences and the Law* 17, no. 4 (1999): 517–41; Lilienfeld, Scott O., Julia Marshall, James T. Todd, and Howard C Shane, "The Persistence of Fad Interventions in the Face of Negative Scientific Evidence: Facilitated Communication for Autism as a Case Example," *Evidence-Based Communication Assessment and Intervention* 8, no. 2 (2014): 62–101, 67–68.

82. Biklen, *Communication Unbound*, 134; Biklen and Duchan, "I Am Intelligent," 182.

83. Trader and Edwards, "Continued Debate," 2.

84. "TASH Resolution on the Right to Communicate," March 2016, https://tash.org/about/resolutions/tash-resolution-right-communicate-2016; Singer, George H. S., Robert H. Horner, Glen Dunlap, and Mian Wang, "Standards of Proof: TASH, Facilitated Communication, and the Science-Based Practices Movement," *Research and Practice for Persons with Severe Disabilities* 39, no. 3 (2014): 178–88, 180.

85. Horner, Robert H., "Facilitated Communication: Keeping It Practical," *Journal of the Association for Persons with Severe Handicaps* 19, no. 3 (1994): 185–86; Singer et al, "Standards of Proof," 178.

86. Salvy, Sarah-Jeanne, James A. Mulick, Eric Butter, Rita Kahng Bartlett, and Thomas R. Linscheid, "Contingent Electric Shock (SIBIS) and a Conditioned Punisher Eliminate Severe Head Banging in a Preschool Child," *Behavioral Interventions* 19, no. 1 (2004): 59–72.

87. Jacobs, Emily, "School for the Disabled Won't Stop Electrically Shocking Its Students," *New York Post*, December 18, 2018, https://nypost.com/2018/12/18/school-for-the-disabled-wont-stop-electrically-shocking-its-students; Setty, Ganesh, "Federal Appeals Court Vacates FDA Rule Banning Electric Shock Devices to Treat Self-Harming Behavior," July 16, 2021, https://www.cnn.com/2021/07/16/health/judge-rotenberg-center-appeals-court-ruling/index.html. Originally called the Behavioral Research Institute, the Judge Rotenberg Educational Center was renamed in 1994 to honor a Massachusetts judge who was instrumental in keeping it open.

88. Lilienfeld et al., "Persistence of Fad Interventions," 76–78.

89. "TASH Resolution on the Right to Communicate"; American Speech-Language-Hearing Association, "Position Statement: Facilitated Communication," 2018, https://www.asha.org/policy/ps2018–00352.

90. Sue Rubin is a particularly prominent example, often cited by proponents of FC, of a person who transitioned from FC to independent communication. Cardinal, Donald N., and Mary A. Falvey, "The Maturing of Facilitated Communication: A Means toward Independent Communication," *Research and Practice for Persons with Severe Disabilities* 39, no. 3 (2014): 189–94; Stubblefield, "Sound and Fury."

Chapter 5. Developmental Disabilities and Subspecialization in Pediatrics

1. Halpern, Sydney A., *American Pediatrics: The Social Dynamics of Professionalism, 1880–1980* (Berkeley: University of California Press, 1988), 153.

2. "Executive Committee Meeting of the Section on Children with Disabilities," November 1993, 4, Section on Children with Disabilities Collection (SCWD), American Academy of Pediatrics Archives (AAP); Capute, Arnold, "Proposal for Subspecialty in Developmental Pediatrics, April 1974," 2, Committee on Children with Handicaps, American Academy of Pediatrics, Capute, Arnold (1973–1976) Folder, Box 119A3, Robert E. Cooke Collection (RC), Alan Mason Chesney Medical Archives of the Johns Hopkins Medical Institutions (JHMI).

3. Capute, "Proposal for Subspecialty," 2.

4. Halpern, *American Pediatrics*; Pawluch, Dorothy, *The New Pediatrics: A Profession in Transition* (Piscataway, NJ: Transaction, 1996).

5. Richmond, Julius B., "Child Development: A Basic Science for Pediatrics," *Pediatrics* 39, no. 5 (1967): 649–58, 656.

6. Robert E. Cooke to Arnold J. Capute, April 25, 1974, "Comments on Subcommittee for Subspeciality on Developmental Pediatrics," Capute, Arnold (1973–1976) Folder, Box 119A3 (RC, JHMI).

7. Abbott, Andrew, *The System of Professions: An Essay on the Division of Expert Labor* (Chicago: University of Chicago Press, 1988); Calvert, Jane, "What's Special about Basic Research?," *Science, Technology & Human Values* 31, no. 2 (2006): 199–220.

8. "J.F.K. Institute Aid Named," *Evening Sun* [Baltimore], July 30, 1969, Biofile, Arnold J. Capute Collection (AC), (JHMI).

9. Bruce Shapiro, interview with author, August 19, 2019.

10. Robert E. Cooke, interview by John F. Stewart, March 29, 1968, 21–22, John F. Kennedy Library Oral History Program, https://www.jfklibrary.org/sites/default/files/archives/JFKOH/Cooke%2C%20Robert%20E/JFKOH-REC-01/JFKOH-REC-01-TR.pdf; Jones, Edgar J., "Helping Handicapped Children to Make the Best of It," *Evening Sun* [Baltimore], October 7, 1977, Biofile (AC, JHMI).

11. Pasquale Accardo, interview with author, August 15, 2019.

12. Shapiro, interview.

13. Accardo, interview; Accardo, Pasquale J., and Arnold J. Capute, *The Pediatrician and the Developmentally Delayed Child: A Clinical Textbook on Mental Retardation* (Baltimore: University Park Press, 1979); Capute, Arnold J., and Pasquale J. Accardo, *Developmental Disabilities in Infancy and Childhood* (Baltimore: Paul H. Brookes, 1991), 28–36.

14. Arnold J. Capute to Robert E. Cooke, October 31, 1973; Robert E. Cooke to Arnold J. Capute, November 12, 1973, Capute, Arnold (1973–1976) Folder, Box 119A3 (RC, JHMI).

15. Accardo, interview.

16. Capute and Accardo, *Developmental Disabilities in Infancy*, 1.

17. Capute and Accardo, *Developmental Disabilities in Infancy*, 27–30.

18. Capute and Accardo, *Developmental Disabilities in Infancy*, 1–3.

19. Park, Edwards A., John W. Littlefield, Henry M. Seidel, and Lawrence S. Wissow, *The Harriet Lane Home: A Model and a Gem* (Baltimore: Johns Hopkins University, 2006),

231, 309; Halpern, *American Pediatrics*, 112–25; F. Curt Bennett, interview with author, January 21, 2021.

20. Arnold J. Capute to Robert E. Cooke, February 28, 1974, Capute, Arnold (1973–1976) Folder, Box 119A3 (RC, JHMI); Accardo, interview.

21. Arnold J. Capute to Robert E. Cooke, February 6, 1973, Capute, Arnold (1973–1976) Folder, Box 119A3 (RC, JHMI); "History: American Academy for Cerebral Palsy and Developmental Medicine," http://www.aacpdm.org/about-us/history.

22. Robert E. Cooke to Lawrence Taft, December 6, 1973, Capute, Arnold (1973–1976) Folder, Box 119A3 (RC, JHMI).

23. Capute to Cooke, February 28, 1974.

24. Arnold J. Capute to Robert E. Cooke, November 14, 1973, 2, Capute, Arnold (1973–1976) Folder, Box 119A3 (RC, JHMI).

25. Capute to Cooke, February 28, 1974.

26. Capute, "Proposal for Subspecialty," 1.

27. Robert E. Cooke to Arnold J. Capute, January 18, 1974, Capute, Arnold (1973–1976) Folder, Box 119A3 (RC, JHMI).

28. Committee on Children with Handicaps Minutes, December 1974, 7 (CCWD, AAP).

29. Capute to Cooke, November 14, 1973; April 2, 1975; November 17, 1975, Capute, Arnold (1973–1976) Folder, Box 119A3 (RC, JHMI).

30. Committee on Children with Handicaps Minutes, May 1974 (CCWD, AAP); Arnold J. Capute to Robert E. Cooke, November 22, 1974, Capute, Arnold (1973–1976) Folder, Box 119A3 (RC, JHMI).

31. Committee on Children with Handicaps Minutes, September 1975, 2 (CCWD, AAP); Warren W. Quillian and Robert C. Brownlee to Arnold J. Capute and Lawrence T. Taft, April 19, 1979, provided by Bruce Shapiro, Department of Pediatrics, Johns Hopkins Medicine (JHM).

32. Capute, Arnold J., and Lawrence Taft, "Ad Hoc Committee for Subspecialty Board in Developmental Pediatrics Draft Proposal," November 1975 Revision, 2–3, Capute, Arnold (1973–1976) Folder, Box 119A3 (RC, JHMI).

33. Committee on Children with Handicaps Minutes, September 1975, 2 (CCWD, AAP).

34. Committee on Children with Handicaps Minutes, November 1976, 5 (CCWD, AAP).

35. Committee on Children with Handicaps Minutes, October 1977, 7 (CCWD, AAP).

36. Committee on Children with Handicaps Minutes, October 1977; Committee on Children with Handicaps Minutes, May 1975; MacQueen, John C., "Report to the AAP Committee on Children with Handicaps," May 22, 1975, 4–5 (CCWD, AAP).

37. Pawluch, *New Pediatrics*, 101–2; Halpern, *American Pediatrics*, 111.

38. Quillian and Brownlee to Capute and Taft, April 19, 1979.

39. Committee on Children with Handicaps Minutes, May 1974 (CCWD, AAP); Capute to Cooke November 22, 1974.

40. Capute, "Proposal for Subspecialty", April 1974, 1; Capute and Taft, "Ad Hoc Committee."

41. O'Keefe, Lori, "Two 'New' Subspecialties: Neurodevelopmental Disabilities and Developmental-Behavioral Pediatrics," *AAP News* (April 2002): 188–89, 188; Accardo,

Pasquale J., Arnold J. Capute, and Michael J. Painter, "Neurodevelopmental Disabilities in Child Neurology: The Creation of a New Sub-Board," *Journal of Pediatrics* 136, no. 2 (2000): 266–67.

42. Capute, Arnold J., and Pasquale J. Accardo, "The Future of Child Neurology: Neurodevelopmental Disabilities in Pediatrics," *Journal of Child Neurology* 7, no. 3 (1992): 315–20, 317.

43. Accardo, interview; Nancy Roizen, interview with author, September 20, 2019; Bennett, interview.

44. "Executive Committee Meeting of the Section on Children with Disabilities," October 1992, 2–3 (SCWD, AAP).

45. Robert C. Brownlee to Arnold J. Capute, June 18, 1990, provided by Bruce Shapiro (JHM); Capute, Arnold J., Bruce K. Shapiro, and Pasquale J. Accardo, "Motor Functions: Associated Primitive Reflex Profiles," *Child Neurology & Developmental Medicine* 24, no. 6 (1982): 662–69; Brody, Jane E. "Child Development: Language Takes on New Significance," *New York Times*, May 5, 1987, C1; Accardo, interview.

46. Accardo, interview; Accardo, Pasquale J., Jennifer A. Accardo, and Arnold J. Capute, "A Neurodevelopmental Perspective on the Continuum Developmental Disabilities," in *Capute & Accardo's Neurodevelopmental Disabilities in Infancy and Childhood*, vol. 1, 3rd ed., ed. Pasquale J. Accardo, 3–26. (Baltimore: Paul H. Brookes, 2008).

47. Accardo et al., "Neurodevelopmental Disabilities in Child Neurology," 267; Accardo, interview.

48. Kevles, Bettyann Holtzmann, *Naked to the Bone: Medical Imaging in the 20th Century* (New Brunswick, NJ: Rutgers University Press, 1997); Danziger, Kurt, *Marking the Mind: A History of Memory* (New York: Cambridge University Press, 2008), 234–42.

49. Richmond, "Child Development: A Basic Science," 656; Richmond, Julius B., "Symposium on Behavioral Pediatrics: An Idea Whose Time Has Arrived," *Pediatric Clinics of North America* 22, no. 3 (1975): 517–23; Haggerty, Robert J., Klaus J. Roghmann, and I. Barry Pless, *Child Health and the Community* (New York: John Wiley & Sons, 1975).

50. Accardo, interview.

51. Haggerty, Robert J., and Stanford B. Friedman, "History of Developmental-Behavioral Pediatrics," *Journal of Developmental and Behavioral Pediatrics* 24, no. 1 (2003): S1–S18.

52. Society for Behavioral Pediatrics, "Executive Committee Meeting Minutes," March 14, 1983, 3–4, University of Maryland, Stanford Friedman, Application (2) Folder (B. 190, F. 2486), William T. Grant Foundation Collection (WTG), Rockefeller Archive Center (RAC).

53. Bennett, interview.

54. Society for Behavioral Pediatrics, "Business Meeting Minutes," May 4, 1983, 2, University of Maryland, Stanford Friedman, Application (2) Folder (B. 190, F. 2486) (WTG, RAC).

55. Richmond, Julius B., "Some Observations on the Sociology of Pediatric Education and Practice," *Pediatrics* 23, no. 6 (1959): 1175–78; Richmond, "Child Development: A Basic Science," 656; Richmond, "Symposium on Behavioral Pediatrics."

56. Bennett, interview; Haggerty et al., *Child Health and the Community*; Blackman,

James A., "Notes from the Chair," *Developmental & Behavioral News* 4, no. 1 (1995): 1–2, 2, Section on Developmental and Behavioral Pediatrics Newsletters (SDBPN), (AAP).

57. Wender, Esther, "Summary: Follow-Up Meeting of the Easton Conference on Behavioral Pediatrics," *Journal of Developmental and Behavioral Pediatrics* 7, no. 3 (1986): 150–51; Friedman, Stanford B., "Behavioral Pediatrics: Interaction with Other Disciplines," *Journal of Developmental and Behavioral Pediatrics* 6, no. 2 (1985): 202–7, 204.

58. "Executive Committee Meeting of the Section on Children with Disabilities," November 1993, 4 (SCWD, AAP).

59. Cohen, Herbert J., A Developmental Pediatrician's Perspective," *Journal of Developmental and Behavioral Pediatrics* 6, no. 4 (1985): 212–13, 213.

60. Haggerty and Friedman, "History of Developmental-Behavioral Pediatrics," S12.

61. Bennett, interview.

62. Capute and Accardo, "Future of Child Neurology," 318; Haggerty and Friedman, "History of Developmental-Behavioral Pediatrics," S12.

63. Slaw, Kenneth M., "Special Meeting: Proposed Section on Developmental Disabilities," September 24, 1990, 2 (SCWD, AAP).

64. Slaw, "Special Meeting: Proposed Section," 2.

65. "Executive Committee Meeting Minutes," October 27, 1991 (SCWD, AAP).

66. "Executive Committee Meeting Minutes," October 27, 1991, 3.

67. "Section on Children with Disabilities Minutes," October 14, 1995, 1 (SCWD, AAP); "Section on Children with Disabilities Five Year Review," August 1995, 3 (SCWD, AAP).

68. James Perrin, interview with author, September 9, 2019.

69. "Executive Committee Meeting Minutes," November 2, 1993, 2–4 (SCWD, AAP).

70. James A. Stockman III to Arnold J. Capute, February 3, 1993, provided by Bruce Shapiro, Department of Pediatrics (JHM).

71. Carey, William B., and John H. Kennell, "Update on Certification," *Journal of Developmental and Behavioral Pediatrics* 14, no. 6 (1993): 430–31, 430.

72. Shapiro, interview. I want to thank Dr. Shapiro for arranging for the framed letters to be briefly taken down and scanned so that I could read them.

73. Shonkoff, Jack P., "Reflections on an Emerging Academic Discipline: The Prolonged Gestation of Developmental and Behavioral Pediatrics," *Journal of Developmental and Behavioral Pediatrics* 14, no. 6 (1993): 409–12.

74. Shonkoff, "Reflections on an Emerging Academic Discipline."

75. Quote from Blackman, "Notes from the Chair," 2; Bennett, interview.

76. Sulkes, Stephen, and Agneta Borgstedt, "What Are We Worth? Relative Value Estimates for Developmental/Behavioral Pediatrics," *Developmental & Behavioral News* 4, no. 1 (1995): 4–5 (SDBPN, AAP).

77. Palfrey, Judith S., "Notes from the Chair," *Developmental & Behavioral News* 4, no. 1 (1995): 1–2, 1; Bennett, Forrest C., "Comments from the Incoming President," *Journal of Developmental and Behavioral Pediatrics* 18, no. 2 (1997): 140–41; Coleman, William L., "A Proposal for Coverage of Behavioral-Developmental Pediatric Issues for Inclusion in the Health Care Reform Act," *Developmental & Behavioral News* 3, no. 1 (1994): 9–11, 9 (SDBPN, AAP).

78. "Section on Children with Disabilities Minutes," 2.

79. Gorski, Peter, "Society for Developmental and Behavioral Pediatrics," *Developmental & Behavioral News* 5, no. 1 (1996): 6 (SDBPN, AAP).

80. Gorski, Peter A., "Presidential Address," *Journal of Developmental and Behavioral Pediatrics* 18, no. 2 (1997): 138–40, 139–40.

81. Bennett, interview; Bennett, "Comments from the Incoming President," 140; Iyama, Tina, "Book Review: *Developmental Disabilities in Infancy and Childhood*, Second Edition," *Journal of Developmental and Behavioral Pediatrics* 18, no. 3 (1997): 206–7.

82. Cohen, Herbert J., "Comments on Receiving the 2004 Arnold J. Capute Award," *Committee / Section on Children with Disabilities Newsletter*, February 2005, 17 (SCWD, AAP).

83. Accardo, interview; Roizen, interview; Shapiro, interview.

84. Coleman, William Lord, "From the Chair: The Struggle for Sub-certification and the Opposition We Face," *Developmental & Behavioral News* 7, no. 1 (1998): 1–7, 6 (SDBPN, AAP).

85. Perrin, Ellen, "Update on Board Certification," *Developmental & Behavioral News* 7, no. 1 (1998): 21–22, 21 (SDBPN, AAP).

86. Coleman, William Lord, "Notes from the Chair," *Developmental & Behavioral News* 5, no. 2 (1995): 1–2 (SDBPN, AAP); Perrin, Ellen C., Forrest C. Bennett, and Mark L. Wolraich, "Subspecialty Certification in Developmental-Behavioral Pediatrics: Past and Present Challenges," *Journal of Developmental and Behavioral Pediatrics* 21, no. 2 (2000): 130–32.

87. Accardo et al., "Neurodevelopmental Disabilities in Child Neurology," 267.

88. Kang, Peter B. et al., "The Child Neurology Clinical Workforce in 2015: Report of the AAP / CNS Joint Taskforce," *Neurology* 87, no. 13 (2016): 1384–92; Gilbert, Donald L. et al., "Child Neurology Recruitment and Training: Views of Residents and Child Neurologists from the 2015 AAP / CNS Workforce Survey," *Pediatric Neurology* 66 (2017): 89–95; Gilbert, Donald L. et al., "Child Neurology Residency Program Directors and Program Coordinators 2016 Workforce Survey," *Pediatric Neurology* 79 (2018): 21–27; Bridgemohan, Carolyn et al., "A Workforce Survey on Developmental-Behavioral Pediatrics," *Pediatrics* 141, no. 3 (2018): e20172164; Roizen, interview.

89. Perrin, interview; Bennett, interview.

90. Bennett, interview.

91. Paul Lipkin, interview with author, September 23, 2019; Council on Children with Disabilities et al., "Identifying Infants and Young Children with Developmental Disorders in the Medical Home: An Algorithm for Developmental Surveillance and Screening," *Pediatrics* 118, no. 1 (2006): 405–20.

92. Abbott, *System of Professions*, 86.

93. Accardo, Pasquale J., ed., *Capute & Accardo's Neurodevelopmental Disabilities in Infancy and Childhood*, 3rd ed. (Baltimore: Paul H. Brooke, 2008).

94. Accardo, Pasquale, "Arnoldisms: Medical Aphorisms of Capute of Hopkins," *Clinical Pediatrics* 33, no. 7 (1994): 444–48, 444.

95. Bennett, F. Curt, "American Board of Pediatrics Update," *Developmental and Behavioral News* 10, no. 1 (2001): 7 (SDBPN, AAP); Bennett, interview.

96. Accardo, interview; Bennett, interview.

97. Hogan, Andrew J., *Life Histories of Genetic Disease: Patterns and Prevention in Postwar Medical Genetics* (Baltimore: Johns Hopkins University Press, 2016); Navon,

Daniel, *Mobilizing Mutations: Human Genetics in the Age of the Patient* (Chicago: University of Chicago Press, 2019).

98. Ralph Amato, interview with author, May 2, 2018; Bruce Buehler, interview with author, November 17, 2017.

99. Before the Human Genome Project, medical genetics held much less prestige and was widely viewed as a backwater in medicine and the biological sciences. Bosk, Charles, *All God's Mistakes: Genetic Counseling in a Pediatric Hospital* (Chicago: University of Chicago Press, 1992); Lindee, Susan, *Moments of Truth in Genetic Medicine* (Baltimore: Johns Hopkins University Press, 2005); Comfort, Nathaniel, *The Science of Human Perfection: Heredity and Health in American Biomedicine* (New Haven, CT: Yale University Press, 2012).

100. McNamara, Elizabeth, "Obituary: Siegfried Max Pueschel," September 4, 2013, https://patch.com/rhode-island/eastgreenwich/amp/18134511/obitu; Pueschel, Siegfried M., "Christian 'Chris' Pueschel (1965–1998)," 1998, https://www.findagrave.com/memorial/31938817/christian-pueschel; Allen Crocker, interview with Julia Heskel, September 26, 2006, Boston Children's Hospital Archives.

101. Crocker, interview; Marquard, Bryan, "Dr. Allen Crocker, 85, Offered Care and Hope to Children with Down Syndrome," *Boston Globe*, November 18, 2011.

102. Rubin, I. Leslie, "Tribute to the Pediatrician Allen C. Crocker (1925–2011)," *International Journal on Disability and Human Development* 11, no. 4 (2012): 295–99, 298; Crocker, interview; Marquard, "Dr. Allen Crocker"; Massachusetts Down Syndrome Congress, "A Tribute to Dr. Allen C. Crocker," September 26, 2011, https://www.youtube.com/watch?v=OougiDvdU-U

103. Brian Skotko, interview with author, July 8, 2019.

104. Crocker, interview.

105. Crocker, Allan C., "Remarks from the Incoming President," *Journal of Developmental and Behavioral Pediatrics* 8, no. 5 (1987): 253–54.

106. Crocker, Allen C., "Presidential Farewell Remarks: 'The Poetry of Childhood,'" *Journal of Developmental and Behavioral Pediatrics* 9, no. 6 (1988): 321–25.

107. Levine, Melvin D., William B. Carey, and Allen C. Crocker, *Developmental-Behavioral Pediatrics* (Philadelphia: W.B. Saunders, 1983); Levine, Melvin D., William B. Carey, and Allen C. Crocker, *Developmental-Behavioral Pediatrics*, 2nd ed. (Philadelphia: W.B. Saunders, 1992), 786.

108. Crocker, Allan C., and Bruce Cushna, "Pediatric Decisions in Children with Serious Mental Retardation," *Pediatric Clinics of North America* 19, no. 2 (1972): 413–21, 415; Crocker, Allan, "Exceptionality," *Journal of Developmental and Behavioral Pediatrics* 19, no. 4 (1998): 300–305.

109. Lippman, Abby, and Benjamin S. Wilfond, "Twice-Told Tales: Stories about Genetic Disorders," *American Journal of Human Genetics* 51, no. 4 (1992): 936–37; Brasington, Campbell K., "What I Wish I Knew Then . . . Reflections from Personal Experiences in Counseling about Down Syndrome," *Journal of Genetic Counseling* 16, no. 6 (2007): 731–34; Wilfond, Benjamin S., "Tracheostomies and Assisted Ventilation in Children with Profound Disabilities: Navigating Family and Professional Values," *Pediatrics* 133, Supplement 1 (2014): S44–S49.

Chapter 6. Keeping the Conversation Open

1. Lippman, Abby, and Benjamin S. Wilfond, "Twice-Told Tales: Stories about Genetic Disorders," *American Journal of Human Genetics* 51, no. 4 (1992): 936–37, 936.

2. Comfort, Nathaniel, *The Science of Human Perfection: Heredity and Health in American Biomedicine* (New Haven, CT: Yale University Press, 2012); Stern, Alexandra Minna, *Telling Genes: The Story of Genetic Counseling in America* (Baltimore: Johns Hopkins University Press, 2012); Hogan, Andrew J., *Life Histories of Genetic Disease: Patterns and Prevention in Postwar Medical Genetics* (Baltimore: Johns Hopkins University Press, 2016).

3. Hogan, *Life Histories of Genetic Disease*; Resta, Robert G., "Historical Aspects of Genetic Counseling: Why Was Maternal Age 35 Chosen as the Cut-Off for Offering Amniocentesis?," *Medicina nei Secoli Art e Scienza* 14, no. 3 (2002): 793–811.

4. National Society of Genetic Counselors, "Professional Status Survey 2020: Executive Summary," 8, https://www.nsgc.org/Policy-Research-and-Publications/Professional-Status-Survey.

5. Begleiter, Michael L., Deborah L. Collins, and Karen Greendale, "NSGC Professional Status Survey," *Perspectives in Genetic Counseling* 3, no. 4 (1981): 1–2, 1; Uhlmann, Wendy R., "Professional Status Survey Results," *Perspectives in Genetic Counseling* 14, no. 2 (1992): 7–10, 7. *Perspectives in Genetic Counseling* available at: https://perspectives.nsgc.org/.

6. Rolnick, Beverly R., "The State of the Society: Remarks to the Annual Business Meeting of the National Society of Genetic Counselors, Inc.," *Perspectives in Genetic Counseling* 3, no. 4 (1981): 4–5, 4.

7. Widmann, Judith D., "Correspondence: To the Editor," *Perspectives in Genetic Counseling* 7, no. 4 (1985): 3.

8. Magyari, Trish, "'Pro-Choice' Update," *Perspectives in Genetic Counseling* 9, no. 1 (1987): 2–3, 2; Magyari, Trish, and Robin Belsky Gold, "Social Issues: Membership Defined by Committee Survey Results," *Perspectives in Genetic Counseling* 10, no. 4 (1988): 1–4, 4.

9. Fitzgerald, Joan, "Letters to the Editor: Semantics and State Legislatures," *Perspectives in Genetic Counseling* 14, no. 4 (1992): 10; Weinblatt, Vivian J., "Letters to the Editor: Professional Roles vs. Personal Beliefs," *Perspectives in Genetic Counseling* 15, no. 1 (1993): 14.

10. Asch, Adrienne, "The Human Genome and Disability Rights: Thoughts for Researchers and Advocates," *Disability Studies Quarterly* 13, no. 3 (1993): 3–4.

11. Cooley, W. Carl, Elizabeth S. Graham, John B. Moeschler, and John M. Graham Jr., "Reactions of Mothers and Medical Professionals to a Film about Down Syndrome," *American Journal of Diseases of Childhood* 144, no. 10 (1990): 1112–16.

12. Marsha Saxton, interview with author, July 13, 2018.

13. Saxton, interview; Saxton, Marsha, "Born and Unborn: The Implications of Genetic Technologies for People with Disabilities," in *Test-Tube Women: What Future for Motherhood?*, ed. Rita Arditti, Renate Duelli Klein, and Shelley Minden, 298–312 (London: Pandora Press, 1984), 308.

14. Saxton, Marsha, "Disability Feminism Meets DNA: A Study of an Educational Model for Genetic Counseling Students on the Social and Ethical Issues of Selective Abortion," (PhD diss., Union Institute, 1996).

15. "Program History," Graduate Program in Genetic Counseling, Brandeis University, http://www.bio.brandeis.edu/genetic-counseling/index.php/the-history-of-the-brandeis -program/.

16. Stern, *Telling Genes*, 94–95.

17. Judith Tsipis, interview with author, July 23, 2018; Zola, Irving Kenneth, *Missing Pieces: A Chronicle of Living with a Disability* (Philadelphia: Temple University Press, 1982).

18. Stern, *Telling Genes*, 175.

19. Saxton, interview; Disability Rights in Dialogue with Clinical Genetics conference, May 31–June 2, 1996, Boston; "Readings on Prenatal Diagnosis and Selective Abortion" (Chicago: Rehabilitation Institute of Chicago, 1996). Provided by Marsha Saxton.

20. Biesecker, Barbara B., Lisa Chen, Jamie Israel, Beth Fine, and Ilana Mittman, "Seeking Common Ground: Dialogue between Disability Rights and Genetics," *Perspectives in Genetic Counseling* 18, no. 3 (1996): 1–8, 8.

21. Asch, Adrienne, "Why I Haven't Changed My Mind about Prenatal Diagnosis: Reflections and Refinements," in *Prenatal Testing and Disability Rights*, ed. Erik Parens and Adrienne Asch, 234–36 (Washington, DC: Georgetown University Press, 2000).

22. Parens, Erik, and Adrienne Asch, "Disability Rights Critique of Prenatal Genetic Testing: Reflections and Recommendations," *Mental Retardation and Developmental Disabilities Research Reviews* 9, no. 1 (2003): 40–47, 42.

23. "Prenatal Testing for Genetic Disability: Meeting IV, October 23–24, 1997," 15, 1997 Prenatal Folder, Box 166, Hastings Center Collection (HCC) 2006–20, National Library of Medicine Archives (NLM).

24. "Prenatal Testing for Genetic Disability: Meeting IV," 18.

25. Kuhse, Helga, and Peter Singer, "Ethics and the Handicapped Newborn Infant," *Social Research* 52, no. 3 (1985): 505–42; Botkin, Jeffrey R., "Line Drawing: Developing Professional Standards for Prenatal Diagnostic Services," in *Prenatal Testing and Disability Rights*, ed. Erik Parens and Adrienne Asch, 288–307 (Washington, DC: Georgetown University Press, 2000); Wertz, Dorothy C., "Drawing Lines: Notes for Policymakers," in *Prenatal Testing and Disability Rights*, ed. Erik Parens and Adrienne Asch, 261–87 (Washington, DC: Georgetown University Press, 2000); Buchanan, Allen, Dan W. Brock, Norman Daniels, and Daniel Wikler, *From Chance to Choice: Genetics and Justice* (Cambridge: Cambridge University Press, 2000); Asch, Adrienne, "Disability, Bioethics, and Human Rights," in *Handbook of Disability Studies*, ed. Gary L. Albrecht, Katherine D. Seelman, and Michael Bury, 297–326 (Thousand Oaks, CA: Sage Publications, 2001); Wasserman, David, "A Choice of Evils in Prenatal Testing," *Florida State University Law Review* 30, no. 1 (2002): 295–313.

26. Parens, Erik, and Adrienne Asch, "Special Supplement: The Disability Rights Critique of Prenatal Genetic Testing Reflections and Recommendations," *Hastings Center Report* 29, no. 5 (1999): S1–S22, S18–S19; Parens, Erik, and Adrienne Asch, eds., *Prenatal Testing and Disability Rights* (Washington, DC: Georgetown University Press, 2000).

27. Barbara Biesecker, interview with author, July 25, 2018; John C. Carey, interview with author, August 12, 2019.

28. Benjamin Wilfond, interview with author, May 16, 2019.

29. Cooke, Robert E., "Whose Suffering," *Journal of Pediatrics* 80, no. 5 (1972): 906–8; Wilfond, Benjamin S., "Tracheostomies and Assisted Ventilation in Children with Pro-

found Disabilities: Navigating Family and Professional Values," *Pediatrics* 133, Supplement 1 (2014): S44–S49.

30. Saxton, interview.

31. Barbara Biesecker, "How Have Similar Sort of Inquiries Fared at NIH?," Planning Meeting Summary Notes, Prenatal Testing for Genetic Disability: Core Consultants Group Meeting #1, June 6, 1996, 1–2, 1996 Prenatal Folder, Box 159. (HCC, NLM).

32. Biesecker, Barbara B., and Lori Hamby, "What Difference the Disability Community Arguments Should Make for the Delivery of Prenatal Genetic Information," in *Prenatal Testing and Disability Rights*, ed. Erik Parens and Adrienne Asch, 340–57 (Washington, DC: Georgetown University Press, 2000), 349.

33. Brasington, Campbell K., "What I Wish I Knew Then . . . Reflections from Personal Experiences in Counseling about Down Syndrome," *Journal of Genetic Counseling* 16, no. 6 (2007): 731–34, 734 (n. 34).

34. Kathryn Peters, interview with author, July 31, 2018.

35. Madeo, Anne C., Barbara B. Biesecker, Campbell Brasington, Lori H. Erby, and Kathryn F. Peters, "The Relationship between the Genetic Counseling Profession and the Disability Community: A Commentary," *American Journal of Medical Genetics Part A* 155, no. 8 (2011): 1777–85, 1781.

36. Dent, Karen M., C. Harper, L. Kearney, C. Lieber, and B. Finucane, "Embracing the Unique Role of Genetic Counselors: Response to the Commentary by Madeo et al.," *American Journal of Medical Genetics Part A* 155, no. 8 (2011): 1791–93, 1792.

37. Bauer, Patricia E., "Reaching across the Disability Divide: The Case for Collaboration with the Disability Community to Construct a Robust Informed Consent Process around Prenatal Screening and Diagnosis," *American Journal of Medical Genetics Part A* 155, no. 8 (2011): 1788–90, 1789.

38. Resta, Robert, "Are Genetic Counselors Just Misunderstood? Thoughts on 'The Relationship between the Genetic Counseling Profession and the Disability Community: A Commentary,'" *American Journal of Medical Genetics Part A* 155, no. 8 (2011): 1786–87, 1786.

39. Sheets, Kathryn B. et al., "Practice Guidelines for Communicating a Prenatal or Postnatal Diagnosis of Down Syndrome: Recommendations of the National Society of Genetic Counselors," *Journal of Genetic Counseling* 20, no. 5 (2011): 432–41; Finucane, Brenda, "Introduction to the Special Issue on Developmental Disabilities," *Journal of Genetic Counseling* 21, no. 6 (2012): 749–51; Hodgson, Jan, and Jon Weil, "Talking about Disability in Prenatal Genetic Counseling: A Report of Two Interactive Workshops," *Journal of Genetic Counseling* 21, no. 1 (2012): 17–23.

40. Lenihan, Melissa, "The Road Less Traveled: One Genetic Counselor's Reflections on Disability and the Genetic Counseling Profession," *Journal of Genetic Counseling* 21, no. 6 (2012): 784–86, 784–85.

41. Farrelly, Ellyn et al., "Genetic Counseling for Prenatal Testing: Where Is the Discussion about Disability?," *Journal of Genetic Counseling* 21, no. 6 (2012): 814–24, 821–22.

42. Hercher, Laura, "Understanding What's Difficult about 'Understanding a Down Syndrome Diagnosis,'" *DNA Exchange*, March 30, 2011, https://thednaexchange.com /2011/03/30/understanding-whats-difficult-about-understanding-a-down-syndrome

-diagnosis/; Kline, Laura, "Disability Awareness Training and Implications for Current Practice: A Survey of Genetic Counselors" (master's thesis, Brandeis University, 2012); Sanborn, Erica, and Annette R. Patterson, "Disability Training in the Genetic Counseling Curricula: Bridging the Gap between Genetic Counselors and the Disability Community," *American Journal of Medical Genetics Part A* 164, no. 8 (2014): 1909–15.

43. National Society of Genetic Counselors, "Position Statements: Disability, Revision," December 2017, https://www.nsgc.org/Policy-Research-and-Publications/Position -Statements/Position-Statements/Post/disability.

44. Anne Madeo, interview with author, August 7, 2019.

45. Hercher, "Understanding What's Difficult."

46. American College of Obstetricians and Gynecologists, "ACOG Practice Bulletin No. 77: Screening for Fetal Chromosomal Abnormalities," *Obstetrics & Gynecology* 109, no. 1 (2007): 217–27.

47. Janice Edwards, interview with author, August 6, 2019.

48. Brasington, "What I Wish I Knew Then."

49. Edwards, interview.

50. Edwards, Janice G., and Richard R. Ferrante, "Toward Concurrence: Understanding Prenatal Screening and Diagnosis of Down Syndrome from the Health Professional and Advocacy Community Perspectives," June 17, 2009, University of South Carolina Center for Disability Resources and Genetic Counseling Program, 2–4, https://www .geneticcounselingtoolkit.com/pdf_files/ConsensusConversationStatement.pdf.

51. Campbell Brasington, interview with author, August 24, 2018; Edwards, interview.

52. Skotko, Brian G., George T. Capone, and Priya S. Kishnani, "Postnatal Diagnosis of Down Syndrome: Synthesis of the Evidence on How Best to Deliver the News," *Pediatrics* 124, no. 4 (2009): e751–58; Skotko, Brian G., Priya S. Kishnani, and George T. Capone, "Prenatal Diagnosis of Down Syndrome: How Best to Deliver the News," *American Journal of Medical Genetics Part A* 149, no. 11 (2009): 2361–67.

53. Skotko, Brian G., "What Would Allen Think Now?," Brian Skotko blog, November 12, 2012, http://brianskotko.com/what-would-allen-think-now/.

54. Stephanie Meredith, interview with author, August 19, 2019; Skotko, Brian G., "Mothers of Children with Down Syndrome Reflect on their Postnatal Support," *Pediatrics* 115, no. 1 (2005): 64–77, 76; Sheets, Katherine Barrier, "Defining Essential Information in a Balanced Description of Down Syndrome" (master's thesis, University of South Carolina, 2009).

55. Leach, Mark W., "The Down Syndrome Information Act: Balancing the Advances of Prenatal Testing through Public Policy," *Intellectual and Developmental Disabilities* 54, no. 2 (2016): 84–93, 84–85; United States Congress, Prenatally and Postnatally Diagnosed Conditions Awareness Act, Public Law 110-374.

56. Brian Skotko, interview with author, July 8, 2019.

57. Skotko, interview.

58. Hogan, Andrew J., "Set Adrift in the Prenatal Diagnostic Marketplace: Analyzing the Role of Users and Mediators in the History of a Medical Technology," *Technology and Culture* 54, no. 1 (2013): 62–89; Mozersky, Jessica, "Hoping Someday Never Comes: Deferring Ethical Thinking about Noninvasive Prenatal Testing," *AJOB Empirical Bioethics* 6,

no. 1 (2015): 31–41; Thomas, Gareth M., Barbara Katz Rothman, Heather Strange, and Joanna Latimer, "Testing Times: The Social Life of Non-Invasive Prenatal Testing," *Science, Technology, and Society* 26, no. 1 (2021): 81–97.

59. Skotko, interview; Hennessey, Matthew, "The Down Syndrome Community's Abortion Rift," *First Things*, November 29, 2012, https://www.firstthings.com/web-exclusives/2012/11/the-down-syndrome-communitys-abortion-rift.

60. *Prenatal Testing & Information about Down Syndrome* (Global Down Syndrome Foundation and National Down Syndrome Congress, 2017), 3, https://www.globaldown syndrome.org/prenatal-testing-pamphlet/.

61. Skotko, "What Would Allen Think Now?"

62. Leach, "Down Syndrome Information Act," 87.

63. Leach, Mark W., "Pro-Life Should Not Hijack Pro-Information," Down Syndrome Prenatal Testing website, January 21, 2015, http://www.downsyndromeprenataltesting.com/pro-life-should-not-hijack-pro-information/; Meredith, interview.

64. Perry, David M., "Anti-Choice Legislators Try to Force Wedge between Reproductive, Disability Rights Activists," *Rewire News Group*, January 16, 2015, https://rewire.news/article/2015/01/16/anti-choice-legislators-try-force-wedge-reproductive-disability-rights-activists/; Perry, David M., "Republicans Are Using Fear of Eugenics to Attack Reproductive Rights," *The Nation*, January 4, 2018, https://www.thenation.com/article/archive/republicans-are-using-fear-of-eugenics-to-attack-reproductive-rights/.

65. Meredith, interview; *Understanding A Down Syndrome Diagnosis* (Lexington: University of Kentucky, 2017), 6–7, 22. Provided by Stephanie Meredith.

66. Wilfond, interview; Bucciarelli, R. L., and Donald V. Eitzman, "Baby Doe: Where We Stand Now," *Contemporary Pediatrics* 5, no. 1 (1988): 116–28; Kopelman, Loretta M., "Are the 21-Year-Old Baby Doe Rules Misunderstood or Mistaken?," *Pediatrics* 115, no. 3 (2005): 797–801.

67. McArdle, Mairead, "Pennsylvania Governor Vetoes Bill Banning Down-Syndrome Abortion," *National Review*, November 22, 2019, https://www.nationalreview.com/news/pennsylvania-governor-vetoes-bill-banning-down-syndrome-abortion/.

68. Allyse, Megan et al., "Non-Invasive Prenatal Testing: A Review of International Implementation and Challenges," *International Journal of Women's Health* 7 (2015): 113–26; Heuvel, Amanda van den et al., "Will the Introduction of Non-Invasive Prenatal Diagnostic Testing Erode Informed Choices? An Experimental Study of Health Care Professionals," *Patient Education* 78, no. 1 (2010): 24–28; Norton, Mary E., Nancy C. Rose, and Peter Benn, "Noninvasive Prenatal Testing for Fetal Aneuploidy: Clinical Assessment and a Plea for Restraint," *Obstetrics & Gynecology* 121, no. 4 (2013): 847–50.

69. Ellyn Farrelly, interview with author, February 26, 2019.

Epilogue

1. This chapter's first three paragraphs draw from several interviews that I conducted with disabled clinicians and other disability advocates. The podcast series Docs with Disabilities offers similar narratives of challenges and successes: https://medicine.umich.edu/dept/family-medicine/programs/mdisability/transforming-medical-education/docs-disabilities-podcast.

2. Asch, Adrienne, "The Experience of Disability: A Challenge for Psychology," *American Psychologist* 39, no. 5 (1984): 529–36; Longmore, Paul K., and Lauri Umansky, *The New Disability History: American Perspectives* (New York: New York University Press, 2001).

3. Engel, George L., "The Need for a New Medical Model: A Challenge for Biomedicine," *Science* 196, no. 4286 (1977): 129–36; Barnes, Colin, "Extended Review," *Disability and Society* 18, no. 6 (2003): 827–33; Hogan, Andrew J., "Social and Medical Models of Disability and Mental Health: Evolution and Renewal," *CMAJ* 191 (2019): E16–E18.

4. Gill, Carol J., "Four Types of Integration in Disability Identity Development," *Journal of Vocational Rehabilitation* 9, no. 1 (1997): 39–46; Hogan, Andrew J., "Moving away from the 'Medical Model': The Development and Revision of the World Health Organization's Classification of Disability," *Bulletin of the History of Medicine* 93, no. 2 (2019): 241–69; Forber-Pratt, Anjali J., Carlyn O. Mueller, and Erin E. Andrews, "Disability Identity and Allyship in Rehabilitation Psychology: Sit, Stand, Sign, and Show Up," *Rehabilitation Psychology* 64, no. 2 (2019): 119–29; Andrews, Erin E. et al., "#SaytheWord: A Disability Culture Commentary on the Erasure of 'Disability,'" *Rehabilitation Psychology* 64, no. 2 (2019): 111–18; Andrews, Erin E., *Disability as Diversity: Developing Cultural Competence* (New York: Oxford University Press, 2020).

5. Hogan, "Moving away from the 'Medical Model.'" The "hidden curriculum" of medical education is a useful concept for examining some of the origins of thinking and practices along the lines of the so-called medical model. Hafferty, Frederic W., "Beyond Curriculum Reform: Confronting Medicine's Hidden Curriculum," *Academic Medicine* 73, no. 4 (1998): 403–7; Piemonte, Nicole, "Last Laughs: Gallows Humor and Medical Education," *Journal of Medical Humanities* 36, no. 4 (2015): 375–90.

6. Abbott, Andrew, *The System of Professions: An Essay on the Division of Expert Labor* (Chicago: University of Chicago Press, 1988).

7. Kuhse, Helga, and Peter Singer, "Ethics and the Handicapped Newborn Infant," *Social Research* 52, no. 3 (1985): 505–42; Parens, Erik, and Adrienne Asch, eds., *Prenatal Testing and Disability Rights* (Washington, DC: Georgetown University Press, 2000); Botkin, Jeffrey R., "Line Drawing: Developing Professional Standards for Prenatal Diagnostic Services," in *Prenatal Testing and Disability Rights*, edited by Erik Parens and Adrienne Asch, 288–307 (Washington, DC: Georgetown University Press, 2000); Wertz, Dorothy C., "Drawing Lines: Notes for Policymakers," in *Prenatal Testing and Disability Rights*, ed. Erik Parens and Adrienne Asch, 261–87 (Washington, DC: Georgetown University Press, 2000); Buchanan, Allen, Dan W. Brock, Norman Daniels, and Daniel Wikler, *From Chance to Choice: Genetics and Justice* (Cambridge: Cambridge University Press, 2000); Asch, Adrienne, "Disability, Bioethics, and Human Rights," in *Handbook of Disability Studies*, ed. Gary L. Albrecht, Katherine D. Seelman, and Michael Bury, 297–326 (Thousand Oaks, CA: Sage Publications, 2001); Wasserman, David, "A Choice of Evils in Prenatal Testing," *Florida State University Law Review* 30, no. 1 (2002): 295–313.

8. Prescott, Heather Munro, *A Doctor of Their Own: A History of Adolescent Medicine* (Cambridge, MA: Harvard University Press, 1998).

9. Lund, Emily M., Rebecca C. Wilbur, and Angela M. Kuemmel, "Beyond Legal Obligation: The Role and Necessity of the Supervisor-Advocate in Creating a Socially Just, Disability-Affirmative Training Environment," *Training and Education in Professional*

Psychology 14, no. 2 (2020): 92–99; Iezzoni, Lisa I., "Why Increasing Numbers of Physicians with Disability Could Improve Care for Patients with Disability," *AMA Journal of Ethics* 18, no. 10 (2016): 1041–49.

10. Shakespeare, Tom, Lisa I. Iezzoni, and Nora E. Groce, "Disability and the Training of Health Professionals," *Lancet* 374 (2009): 1815–16, 1816.

11. Cooper-Patrick, L. et al., "Race, Gender, and Partnership in the Patient-Physician Relationship," *JAMA* 282, no. 6 (1999): 583–89; Bristow, L. R., A. S. Butler, and B. D. Smedley, *In the Nation's Compelling Interest: Ensuring Diversity in the Health-Care Workforce* (Washington, DC: National Academies Press, 2004).

12. Forber-Pratt et al., "Disability Identity and Allyship"; Gill, Carol J., "The Family / Professional Alliance in Rehabilitation Viewed from a Minority Perspective," *American Behavioral Scientist* 28, no. 3 (1985): 424–28; Olkin, Rhoda, *What Psychotherapists Should Know about Disability* (New York: Guilford Press, 1999), 308.

Index

Abbott, Andrew, 7, 153

ableism, 34, 37, 192

abortion, 171–73, 179–80, 191; legislation (restrictive), 162, 181–82; opposition, 69, 162–63; selective, 1, 11, 83, 91, 100, 160–61, 165–68, 175–77, 185, 192; support, 4, 89, 163–64

Accardo, Pasquale, 134–36, 143

adaptive skills (behaviors), in mental retardation assessment, 116–21, 155

advocacy, definition, 4–5. *See also* disability self-advocacy

alternative therapies, 105, 109–11

Amato, Ralph, 92

American Academy of Pediatrics, 58, 60, 68, 70–74, 139, 146–48; Committee on Children with Disabilities (Handicaps), 48–49, 52–53, 59, 62–63, 67–69, 72, 137–40, 145–48, 152; Executive Board, 53; medical home, 71–75, 148; Section on Children with Disabilities, 141, 146–49, 152; Section on Developmental and Behavioral Pediatrics, 146, 149, 151, 153

American Association on Intellectual and Developmental Disabilities, 106

American Association on Mental Deficiency, 6, 48, 105

American Association on Mental Retardation, 106; Board of Directors (executive board), 105, 110–11; positions on aversives, 105, 109–11, 114; terminology and classification manual, 115–22

American Board of Genetic Counseling, 92

American Board of Medical Genetics, 97, 156

American Board of Medical Specialties, 133, 151, 156

American Board of Pediatrics, 131, 138–42, 148, 151

American Board of Psychiatry and Neurology, 142, 150

American College of Medical Genetics, 176. *See also* medical genetics

American College of Obstetricians and Gynecologists, 175

American Medical Association, 61

American Psychological Association, 19–35, 115; Board of Social and Ethical Responsibility for Psychology, 30; Committee on Disabilities and Handicaps, 27–28; Committee on Ethics 19, 30, 45; Division 33, 106–7, 117, 128–29

Americans with Disabilities Act, 10, 29–32, 34–35, 189, 191

amniocentesis, 83, 162, 175, 179, 183

Andrews, Erin, 15, 34–36

Asch, Adrienne: background, 26, 164; genetic counseling, 98–100, 164, 167–70; psychology, 26–27, 29

Association of University Affiliated Facilities, 60

augmentative and alternative communication technologies, 127–28

autism, 7, 105, 111–12, 122–24, 126, 135–36, 147, 149

aversives, 105–14; ongoing use, 128–29

Baby Doe Rules, 70, 182, 191

Barker, Roger G., 22–23

basic (science) research, 53–55, 94, 132, 144

Battle, Constance, 64–65, 72

Battle, Ursula, 64

Beaven, Paul, 52–53

behavior modification, 106–8, 111–12

behavioral pediatrics. *See* developmental and behavioral pediatrics

Benkendorf, Judith, 96

Bennett, F. Curt, 150

Bennett, Robin, 82–83

Biesecker, Barbara, 93, 96, 100–101, 169–72

Biklen, Douglas, 122–25, 129

bioethics, 12, 36, 90, 167–69; focus in severity, 12, 69, 112, 168, 192

biopsychosocial model, 14, 150, 190

Bosk, Charles, 82

Boston Children's Hospital, 65–66, 148, 157

brain damage, chronic (organic), 17, 135–36, 140–43, 147–48, 154, 186